Gestational Diabetes Food List

100 Recipes for Balanced Energy and Healthy Pregnancy

Kate Princeton Johnson

Table of Contents

Introduction

Pregnancy is one of the greatest miracles of life. It is difficult to comprehend how something microscopically tiny can grow for 40 week into a tiny human being inside your body! 'Enjoy the journey," is perhaps one of the most common pieces of advice you are going to receive from women who have been there.

A radiant glow is one of pregnancies most looked forward to gift. But, of course even this can be a little clouded by a few less pleasant 'side effects'. But, as you'll soon learn, you won't even have time to bemoan a few inconveniences especially when you consider the fact that your body is performing one of the most important miracles of nature.

Now, a very important thing that you should be well aware of as you prepare to get pregnant or as you start to enjoy this beautiful journey is gestational diabetes. This is a type of diabetes that first manifests itself during pregnancy. Once you deliver your baby, gestational diabetes usually disappears.

However, before we move any further into the topic, I know that this diagnosis can literally turn everything upside down, especially if this is your first time hearing about gestational diabetes. Your first instinct will be to worry about how your child is going to be affected and whether you will have to be on insulin shots and what these will mean for your unborn baby.

But, I am here to quell all your fears and provide you with information that is going to help you embrace a healthy lifestyle by tweaking your diet.

We are going to delve deeper into gestational diabetes in a bid to understand what causes it, what does it mean for you, whether it affects the baby, who is at risk, what you should do if diagnosed with it. So, let's get started!

What Causes Gestational Diabetes?

Gestational diabetes occurs when a woman who has not been previously diagnosed with diabetes develops significantly high blood sugar levels in the course of her pregnancy. We understand that there are a lot of hormonal changes that take place when you become pregnant and one of the hormones that can get affected is insulin. Insulin is tasked with keeping your blood sugar levels at steady and healthy levels.

When pregnant, the interaction of other hormones can obstruct your body's sensitivity to insulin causing your blood sugar levels to become elevated.

The best part of gestational diabetes is that it usually disappears on its own after delivery with blood sugars stabilizing.

Now, the question that most people ask is, if gestational diabetes disappears right after delivery, then what's the big deal?

The biggest problem with gestational diabetes is that the mother ends up having spiked sugar levels that are able to pass through the placenta to the unborn baby.

For most women, once gestational diabetes is diagnosed they are going to be provided with proper care and advice during prenatal doctor visits.

However, a few complications could arise for the baby, if not properly managed, such as jaundice, low blood sugar levels at birth, low calcium levels and breathing problems. Additionally, high blood sugar levels in the mother could lead to macrosimia which is when a fetus grows much bigger than normal , an excess of amniotic fluid being produced or in extreme cases, a still birth. Preeclampsia and high blood pressure are other possible risks associated with gestational diabetes.

So, in as much as it will reverse on its own, the effects on [pregnancy and birth can be quite serious.

How Is Gestational Diabetes Diagnosed?

Many women with gestational diabetes do not have easily identifiable symptoms. Most will experience thirst, hunger and fatigue, which are normal symptoms of pregnancy.

You may think that by leading a generally healthy lifestyle of eating whole, natural and healthy foods and exercising on a regular basis that you can't get gestational diabetes but it's not a guarantee.

This is not to mean that you should throw all caution to the wind and start eating anything you crave even when it's not healthy. Remember, that what you eat is also what nourishes your baby and so it's important that you tweak your diet o include foods that are rich in vitamins, minerals and nutrients that are good for both you and the baby

It is important to get tested between your 24th and 28th week of pregnancy. The test is usually a one hour glucose tolerance test. If this turns positive, you are given a three hour glucose tolerance test just to confirm that you actually have gestational diabetes.

Common symptoms of gestational diabetes

- Excess fatigue
- Very frequent yeast infections
- Extreme thirst
- Abnormally frequent urination

Real Food for Gestational Diabetes

The recipes provided in this book and the concepts herein are based on natural, real and healthy foods. The typical diabetes diet often features sugar-free foods which have been shown to be even more harmful as they feature artificial sweeteners. You will also notice a restrictive carb count without really paying proper attention to the other foods that you are going to be eating.

In this gestational diabetes guide, we are going to focus our attention on real and natural foods that will not only help you balance your blood sugars but that will also provide your unborn baby with the best nutrition for optimal growth.

Our approach focuses on creating a perfect balance of complex carbohydrates, protein and healthy fats that is going to play a pivotal role in controlling your blood sugars. Perhaps the best thing about this guide is that it is not restrictive in as much as we are talking about gestational diabetes. We teach you how to enjoy very healthy meals which will give you the peace of mind of knowing that you and baby are getting the best nutrition you can.

The role of Carbs

As a way of keeping gestational diabetes under control, it's important to note that while it is not all about carbs, out of the three classes of macronutrients, that is, carbs, fats and protein, it's only carbs that cause a spike of your blood sugar.

The first step in controlling blood sugar spikes is in understanding the difference between complex carbs and simple carbs. It is true that not all carbs are created equally.

There are two classes of carbohydrates and they are:

1. Complex carbs

Complex carbs are rich in fiber and dietary starch and come directly from plants without undergoing any refining. They slowly release energy in your body thus keeping you full longer and also help boost your digestive process because of their high fiber content. Most complex carbs are plant based meaning they also nourish your body with potent vitamins antioxidants and minerals.

They consist of:

Great Natural Sources of Complex Carbs

Certain foods are naturally endowed with complex carbohydrates and since many of these are plant based, they are also very rich in antioxidants, minerals and vitamins.

- Whole grains

Whole grains are very high in complex carbs and are commonly used in breads, pastas and rice. It is very important that you know how to differentiate foods made from whole grains and those made from refined grain flours such as white rice, white pasta and white bread. Food made from refined grain flours contains simple carbs that as we saw earlier can result in weight gain and disease.

Whole grains are also rich in fiber which aids in digestions and minerals that support your immune function, natural detoxification process, bone formation and cognitive function.

- Quinoa

Very rich in complex carbs, quinoa is also endowed with protein, B vitamins and magnesium. Quinoa has additionally been shown to significantly lower appetite and boost metabolism which is very helpful if you are looking to shed some weight.

- Fruit

Both complex carbs and simple carbs are found in fruit and while simple carbs are known to have negative effects, the benefits you get from consuming fruit in terms of complex carbs, vitamins, antioxidants and minerals outweigh the negative effects of simple carbs.

If you have a sweet tooth, fruit is the perfect substitute for processed sweets as the sugars found in fruit are natural thus don't cause the sudden spikes and surges of blood sugar as is the case for processed sugars. Prunes and apples are amazing complex carbs sources that also rank low on the glycemic index.

- Legumes

Peas, lentils and beans are not only rich in complex carbs but also protein, fiber, folic acid and potent minerals that boost all your bodily functions. Folic acid is especially beneficial for prenatal care as it helps healthy development of a fetus' DNA.

- Root veggies

Root vegetables get their nutrients by soaking up and absorbing nutrients from the surrounding soil. This way they are endowed with complex carbs and a host of minerals such as potassium and magnesium and vitamins A, C and E. sweet potatoes, parsnips, artichokes, potatoes and onions are very healthy root vegetable options.

- Buckwheat

Commonly associated with the wheat family, buckwheat actually belongs to the pseudo cereal family. Pseudo cereals are seeds that don't grow on grass. Others include amaranth and quinoa. Buckwheat is super rich on complex carbs, fiber, antioxidants and minerals. The fiber contained in buckwheat is not digestible by the body and it's actually very good for the colon. Buckwheat husk also contains resistant starch that's not digestible and is also categorized as fiber.

- Whole-wheat

100 percent whole wheat that contains both the germ and bran of the wheat is an excellent source of complex carbs, magnesium, manganese and dietary fiber. Whole wheat breads, pastas and noodles are more nutritious substitutes of white breads, pastas and noodles.

- Farro,

Farro is packed with complex carbs, protein, fiber and potent minerals. Chewy with a rich flavor profile, farro is an amazing rain to have in your pantry that goes really well with almost every veggie and protein dish.

Other great sources of complex carbs include, non-starchy veggies such as spinach, brussel sprouts and sweet peppers.

2. Simple carbs

These provide your body with the literal 'pick-me-up' energy as they are digested very quickly in your body owing to the fact they are mostly sugar. They are derived from complex carbs which is processed to now produce simple carbs. Unfortunately, this is the type of carbs that we mostly overeat especially since they tend to be really tasty, but for someone with type 2 diabetes or gestational diabetes, they spell doom!

Simple carbs can be found in:

Desserts and pastries made from refined flours and processed sugars, added sugars of all kinds, sugary beverages and refined grains.

For people with type 2 diabetes or gestational diabetes, their daily carbs intake should not exceed 150 rams. This amount has been shown by the Institute of Medicine to be very effective in controlling your blood glucose and to also meet your body's nutrient requirements. However, this value can change based on your age, weight, race, activity level, gestation period and dietary needs. Your nutritionist will help come up with the right amount of carbs you should be eating in a day.

Another great way of determining how much of carbs you should be taking is to closely monitor you blood glucose levels. The best time to check is a few minutes after waking up before you eat anything. If your reading are slightly elevated then you know that your carb intake should be minimal. On the other hand, if your glucose levels are very low, then you know that you need to take slightly more carbs than you normally would.

Understanding What's Going On

Gestational diabetes is generally managed and treated in a very similar way to type 2 diabetes or pre-diabetes and the reason for this is because they are in essence the same thing, that is, it boils down to insulin resistance in each case.

Insulin resistance

Insulin is a hormone that is secreted in the pancreas and tasked with taking out sugar from your blood stream, after digestion, and taking it to cells where it is utilized as energy. Insulin resistance means that your body stops responding to insulin as it should and as such blood sugar levels keep rising and rising which inadvertently triggers your pancreas to release even more insulin to try and balance the high levels of blood sugar.

With time, this becomes normal for your body and it stops responding to insulin as it should and at this point your cells become resistant to insulin.

When we come pregnancy, even without gestational diabetes, the mother's body is naturally triggered by pregnancy to resist insulin. This goes back to the evolution of man where humans did not have frequent meals and had to endure periods of drought and famine. Foods rich in carbs were very scarce and the induction of insulin resistance meant that the mother's body took in very little energy with the rest being directed towards the growing baby. This is a very genius story of survival!

Fast forward many years later and we are now in a world of carbohydrate abundance and this primal adaptive way of life is now working against us. While starvation is not a choice you should contemplate as you need to properly nourish your baby, choosing foods that do not cause a spike in blood sugar levels naturally and avoiding simple carbs that cause blood glucose spikes is the best and most beneficial solution.

As pregnancy advances and the mother's body continues to release higher amounts of cortisol, estrogen, progesterone and human placental lactogen, insulin resistance becomes more and more heightened. This is the reason why gestational diabetes is tested at 24 to 28 weeks of pregnancy. this is also the reason why in the third trimester, women who are not able to lower their blood sugar levels naturally need insulin shots or other blood sugar suppressing drugs.

Is your blood sugar normal?

If you are slightly familiar with normal blood sugar levels maybe from family or friends who are diabetic, then you may be in a position to know what's considered low, normal or high. However, this is not exactly the case when it comes to pregnancy reason being that normal blood sugar levels are a little lower than for similar non-pregnant adults.

One of the causes for this is that the blood of a pregnant woman is slightly lighter or diluted because of the increased amount of fluid in the circulatory system. This extra fluid leads to the dilution of blood glucose as well.

- Fasting testing

This is the blood sugar reading that you take first thing when you wake up before you take your breakfast or any food that has caloric value. The normal blood sugar level for pregnancy when fasting is about 90mg/dl.

- After- meal testing

This reading is done about an hour after taking your first bite. The normal blood sugar level is about 130mg/dl. The longer you stay before you test after eating, the lower your reading should be. If you do your test 2 hours after eating, your reading should be about 120mg/dl.

Blood sugar levels that are significantly higher than these values can be quite dangerous for your unborn child. Anything above 140mg/dl is termed as very high. This can lead to blood sugar spikes in your baby and cause him. Her to develop insulin resistance which can be quite tasking for their tiny pancreas.

Above 200mg/dl and this is actually dangerous and has been linked to severe structural deformities such as missing limbs and heart defects in unborn babies. However, this extreme case is mostly seen in women who have undiagnosed type 2 diabetes or very poorly managed type 1 diabetes that have uncontrolled blood sugar levels especially in the first 2 months of pregnancy where organ formation begins.

We are now going to look at the best ways to manage gestational diabetes to keep both you and baby safe throughout your pregnancy.

Best Practices to Manage Gestational Diabetes

- Medical support

Medical support from your doctor, nutritionist, and pre-natal care nurse or diabetes specialist is going to be paramount. As a mother, especially if this is your first time being diagnosed with gestational diabetes, it is normal to get super stressed about whether your baby is going to be fine. You need proper support to help keep you calm and stress free to ensure your baby also grows healthy. Having the right information will help you know the exact steps and measures that you are supposed to take.

- Exercise

Unless your doctor has advised that you don't engage in any form of physical exercise, regular, moderate physical activity plays a pivotal role in managing gestational diabetes. This is because it helps stabilize your blood glucose levels by reducing your body's insulin resistance. It's important to keep in mind that engaging in exercise will mean a significant increase in your heart rate and breathing and you should therefore get approval from your midwife or obstetrician before you engage in any form of exercise.

- A healthy and balanced diet

Eating a well-diversified and healthy diet can help you manage your blood sugar levels. For people suffering from diabetes, it's recommended that they eat small, regular meals often. When it comes to carbohydrates, avoid all simple carbohydrates such refined flours, white bread, white rice, white pasta and processed sugars as these cause a spike in blood sugar levels.

- Keep track of your blood glucose levels

As you progress in your pregnancy, it is important that you keep monitoring your blood sugar levels. This will let you know what dietary and lifestyle changes are positively or negatively impacting your gestational diabetes. If you lead a healthy lifestyle of watching what you eat and exercising and are still not able to control your blood sugar, your doctor will prescribe medication to help you out and show you how to take the medicine which could be in the form of an insulin injection.

- Hydrate

Drinking eight glasses of water every day helps your bodily functions to operate well by flushing out toxins.

What Happens After Birth?

If you were on diabetes medication, this will stop after your baby is born, under normal circumstances, and this is attributed to the fact that for most women who have gestational diabetes, blood sugar levels return to normal after delivery.

Something very important to point out is that just because you have gestational diabetes does not mean that your baby is going to be born with diabetes but they have an increased chance of developing type 2 diabetes later in life. Another thing is that it also puts you at an increased risk of getting type 2 diabetes and you should therefore continue watching your diet and eating whole complex carbs in place of simple refined carbs.

Are You At Risk Of Getting Gestational Diabetes?

You may be at risk if:

1. Your family has a history of type 2 diabetes
2. Are 40 years old and above
3. Have had gestational diabetes in previous pregnancies
4. Have delivered a baby weighing 4.5kg and more before
5. Are obese or overweight
6. You have (PCOS) Polycystic Ovarian Syndrome
7. You have experienced complicated pregnancies before

Now that you are equipped with the right information regarding gestation diabetes, you can now move forward confidently knowing what you should do if you have gestational diabetes or if you develop it. Below are tasty recipes designed to help balance and normalize you blood sugar levels. They are not just restricted to gestational diabetes, you can enjoy them long after birth to help you stay healthy and well nourished.

30-Day Gestational Diabetes Meal Plan

Day	Breakfast	AM SNACK	Lunch	PM SNACK	Dinner
Day 1	1 Serving Spiced Omelets with Red Onions & Chilli	Handful Toasted Coconut Flakes	1 Serving Pan-Seared Mackerel Salad with Snow Peas & Grapefruit	1 Serving Turmeric Coconut Latte	1 Serving Pan-Fried Chili Beef with Toasted Cashews
Day 2	1 Serving Spiced Buckwheat Pancakes with Elderberries	1 Serving Healthy Nutty Guacamole	1 Serving Stir-Fried Mushrooms & Spinach with Golden Onions	Handful Blueberries	1 Serving Romaine Lettuce with Caramelized Onions & Grilled Sardines
Day 3	1 Serving Omelets with Greens & Mushrooms	Tahini and Celery	1 Serving Super Cleansing Avocado-Kale Salad with Grilled Lime Steak	1 Serving Bacon-Avocado stuffed Peppers	1 Serving Healthy Keto Coconut-Lime Skirt Steak
Day 4	1 Serving Hot Almond Butter Flax Meal Cereal	1 Serving Delicious Ginger Tahini Dip	1 Serving Beef Stir Fry with Red Onions & Cabbage	1 Green Apple	1 Serving Lemon & Garlic Barbecued Ocean Trout
Day 5	1 Serving Chopped Leftover Salmon with Wilted Spinach & Avocado	Handful Toasted Cashews	1 Serving Scrumptious Beef & Green Bean Stir-Fry	1 Slice Avocado	1 Serving Pepper Crusted Steak

Day 6	1 Serving Antioxidant-Rich Coconut & Blackberry Smoothie Bowl	1 Serving Spiced Tahini Hummus	1 Serving Barbecued Steak Salad with Thai Dressing	Handful Blueberries	1 Serving Barbecued Spiced Salmon with Avocado-Mango Salsa
Day 7	1 Serving Healthy Omelets with Greens & Shiitake Mushrooms	1 Serving Spiced & Sweet Lassi	1 Serving Spicy cauliflower	Handful Toasted Almonds	1 Serving Ground Beef Lettuce Tacos
Day 8	1 Serving Healthy Keto Almond Flour Porridge	1 Serving Roasted Spiced Pumpkin Seeds	1 Serving Steamed Chicken with Mushroom and Ginger	1 Pear	1 Service Pork, Toasted Almonds & Pumpkin with chimichurri
Day 9	1 Serving Ground Beef, Eggs and Avocado Breakfast Bowl	Handful Blueberries	1 Serving Grilled Chicken with Rainbow Salad Bowl	1 Serving Spicy Peanut Masala	1 Serving Delicious Low Carb Chicken Curry
Day 10	1 Serving Low Carb Coconut Flour Pancakes	1 Serving Oven-Roasted Asparagus	1 Serving Grilled Mushrooms Served with Grilled Steak	Handful Toasted Sunflower Seeds	1 Serving Herb & Walnut Crusted Salmon
Day 11	1 Serving Healthy Scallions & Smoked Salmon Frittata	1 Serving Spiced Apple Crisps	1 Serving Charred Chicken with Healthy Broccoli Salad	Handful Blueberries	1 Serving Beef Stir Fry with Red Onions & Cabbage

Day 12	1 Serving Immune Booster Breakfast Muesli	Handful Toasted Almonds	1 Serving Turkey & Coconut Soup	1 Serving Low Carb Pecan Fudge Fat Bombs	1 Serving Pan-Fried Chili Beef with Toasted Cashews
Day 13	1 Serving Pan-Fried Mushrooms, Boiled Eggs, Spinach & Capsicum	1 Serving Roasted Chili-Vinegar Peanuts	1 Serving Low Carb Berry Salad with Citrus Dressing	½ Avocado	1 Serving Stir-Fried Chicken with Water Chestnuts
Day 14	1 Serving Grain-Free Dairy-Free Pancakes	Handful Toasted Coconut Flakes	1 Serving Pepper Beef and Lettuce Wraps	1 Serving Gingery Lemonade	1 Serving Lemon-pepper BBQ fish with greens and salsa
Day 15	1 Serving Curried Egg Frittata	1 Serving Roasted Asparagus	1 Serving Vegetable Detox Soup	1 Pear	1 Serving Healthy Keto Coconut-Lime Skirt Steak
Day 16	1 Serving Spiced Buckwheat Pancakes with Elderberries	Handful Toasted Sesame Seeds	1 Serving Creamy Detox Broccoli Soup	1 Serving Crispy Lemon- Chili Roasted Kale	1 Serving Tilapia with Mushroom Sauce
Day 17	1 Serving Spiced White Fish Breakfast Frittata	1 Serving Healthy Taro Chips	1 Serving Green Salad with Beets & Edamame	Tahini and Celery	1 Serving Delicious Chicken Tikka Skewers
Day 18	1 Serving Healthy Detox Porridge	Handful Toasted Cashews	1 Serving Healthy Lunch Salad with Hot Creamy Avocado Dressing	1 Serving Heart-Healthy Fats Smoothie	1 Serving Healthy Low-Carb Grilled Turkey

Day 19	1 Serving Healthy Avocado Shrimp Omelet	1 Serving Amaranth Pop Corns	1 Serving Tamarind Sauce Fish Curry	Handful Macadamia Nuts	1 Serving Ginger Chicken with Veggies
Day 20	1 Serving Low Carb Berry Shake	Handful Blueberries	1 Serving Vegetable Detox Soup	1 Serving Healthy Seed Crackers	1 Serving Healthy Roast Salmon with Green Salsa
Day 21	1 Serving Spiced Egg Frittata	Handful Toasted Almonds	1 Serving Healthy Detox Salad with Grilled White Fish	1 Serving Lemon Olive Snack	1 Serving Coconut-Crumbed Chicken Bake
Day 22	1 Serving Immune Booster Breakfast Muesli	1 Serving Sugar-Free Peanut Butter Fudge	1 Serving Steamed Chicken with Mushroom and Ginger	1 Pear	1 Serving Hot Lemon Prawns
Day 23	1 Serving Spiced Breakfast Egg Scramble	Handful Blueberries	1 Serving Chicory & orange salad with ginger dressing	1 Serving Spiced Spinach Bites	1 Serving Beef Stir Fry with Red Onions & Cabbage
Day 24	1 Serving Low Carb Coconut Flour Pancakes	1 Serving Sesame Carrots	1 Serving Anti-Inflammatory Spiced Carrot Soup	Handful Toasted Cashews	1 Serving Creamy Coconut Sardines Escabeche
Day 25	1 Serving Avocado and Egg Breakfast	Handful Cacao Nibs	1 Serving Grilled Beef & Steamed Veggie Salad with Macadamia Dressing	1 Serving Sesame Crackers	1 Serving Ground Beef Lettuce Tacos

Day 26	1 Serving Antioxidant-Rich Coconut & Blackberry Smoothie Bowl	1 Serving Tasty Coconut Raspberry Fat Bombs	1 Serving Healthy Salad with Grilled Chicken Wrap	1 Green Apple	1 Serving Tangy Whole Roasted Sea Bass with Oregano
Day 27	1 Serving Low Carb Smoked Salmon Omelet	Handful Toasted Almonds	1 Serving Healthy Lunch Salad with Hot Creamy Avocado Dressing	1 Serving Cashew Butter Fat Bombs	1 Serving Curried Goat Stew
Day 28	1 Serving Hot Almond Butter Flax Meal Cereal	1 Serving Healthy Nutty Guacamole	1 Serving Authentic and Easy Shrimp Curry	Tahini and Celery	1 Serving Ginger Chicken with Veggies
Day 29	1 Serving Spiced White Fish Breakfast Frittata	Handful Blueberries	1 Serving Clean Eating Lemon Grilled Salmon & Avocado Vegetable Salad	1 Serving Easy No Bake Coconut Cookies	1 Serving Lean Steak with Healthy Pistachio Pesto
Day 30	1 Serving Anti-Inflammatory Ginger Almond Blueberry Smoothie Bowl	1 Serving Bacon-Avocado stuffed Peppers	1 Serving Beef Stir Fry with Red Onions & Cabbage	Handful Toasted Coconut Flakes	1 Serving Spiced Roast Side of Salmon

1. Chopped Leftover Salmon with Wilted Spinach & Avocado

Yield: 2 Servings
Total Time: 25 Minutes
Prep Time: 10 Minutes
Cook Time: 15 Minutes

Ingredients

- 2 leftover grilled salmon fillets, chopped
- 1 tablespoon extra-virgin olive oil
- 1/2 pound mushrooms
- 2 cloves garlic
- 2 cups spinach
- 2 tomatoes
- salt and pepper
- 1 tablespoon apple cider vinegar
- 1 tablespoon olive oil
- Avocado, diced

Directions

Heat olive oil in a pan over medium heat; sauté mushrooms, garlic and tomatoes for about 5 minutes or until tender. Add spinach and cook until wilted; season with salt and pepper and transfer the veggies to a plate. Warm your leftover salmon and serve with the veggies drizzled with vinegar and avocado slices on the side.

Nutrition information per Serving:

Calories: 620; Total Fat: 45.3 g; Carbs: 19.3 g; Dietary Fiber: 10.1 g; Sugars: 5.9 g; Protein: 42.1 g; Cholesterol: 78 mg; Sodium: 122 mg

2. Spiced Buckwheat Pancakes with Elderberries

Yield: 4 Servings
Total Time: 26 Minutes
Prep Time: 10 Minutes
Cook Time: 16 Minutes

Ingredients

- 4 tablespoons coconut oil
- 1 cup coconut milk
- 1 cup ground buckwheat flour
- ½ teaspoon chili powder
- ¼ teaspoon turmeric powder
- teaspoon salt
- ¼ teaspoon black pepper
- ½ inch ginger, grated
- 1 serrano pepper, minced
- 1 handful cilantro, chopped
- ½ red onion, chopped
- 1 cup fresh elderberries to serve

Directions

In a bowl, combine coconut milk, buckwheat, and spices until well blended; stir in ginger, Serrano pepper, cilantro, and red onion until well combined.

Melt coconut oil in a saucepan over medium low heat; add about ¼ cup of batter and spread out on the pan.

Cook for about 4 minutes per side or until golden brown. Transfer to a plate and keep warm; repeat with the remaining batter and oil.

Top the pancakes with fresh elderberries and fold into wraps. Serve with a glass of freshly squeezed orange juice.

Nutritional Information per Serving:

Calories: 386; Total Fat: 33.9 g; Carbs: 20.5 g; Dietary Fiber: 3.5g; Sugars: 3.2 g; Protein: 4.1 g; Cholesterol: 0 mg; Sodium: 596 mg

3. Healthy Omelets with Greens & Shiitake Mushrooms

Yield: 2 Servings
Total Time: 25 Minutes
Prep Time: 10 Minutes
Cook Time: 15 Minutes

Ingredients

- 3 egg whites
- 1 egg
- 1/2 teaspoon extra-virgin olive oil
- 1/8 teaspoon red pepper flakes
- 1/8 teaspoon ground nutmeg
- 1/8 teaspoon garlic powder
- 1/4 teaspoon salt
- 1/8 teaspoon ground black pepper
- 1/2 cup sliced fresh shiitake mushrooms
- 2 tablespoons chopped red bell pepper
- 1/4 cup chopped green onion
- 1/2 cup chopped tomato
- 1 cup chopped fresh spinach

Directions

In a large bowl, whisk together egg whites, egg, garlic powder, red pepper flakes, nutmeg, salt and pepper until well blended.
Heat olive oil in a skillet over medium heat; add green onion, mushrooms and belle pepper and cook for about 5 minutes or until tender; stir in tomato and egg mixture and cook for about 5 minutes per side or until egg is set. Slice and serve hot.

Nutrition information per Serving:

Calories: 127; Total Fat: 4 g; Carbs: 13.7 g; Dietary Fiber: 3.1 g; Sugars: 8.4 g; Protein: 11 g; Cholesterol: 82 mg; Sodium: 392 mg

4. Hot Almond Butter Flax Meal Cereal

Yield: 1 Serving
Total Time: 8 Minutes
Prep Time: 5 Minutes
Cook Time: 3 Minutes

Ingredients:

- 1/2 cup flax seed meal
- 1/2 cup boiling water
- 1/4 teaspoon cinnamon
- 1 tablespoon almond butter

Directions

In a pan of water, stir in flax seed meal and cook for about 2 minutes; stir in cinnamon and almond butter and cook for 2 minutes or until thick.
Remove and serve right away.

Nutritional Information per Serving:

Calories: 395; Total Fat: 26.6 g; Carbs: 19.5 g; Dietary Fiber: 17.1 g; Sugars: 1.5 g; Protein: 13.8 g; Cholesterol: 0 mg; Sodium: 21 mg

5. Spiced Omelets with Red Onions & Chilli

Yield: 2 Servings
Total Time: 20 Minutes
Prep Time: 10 Minutes
Cook Time: 10 Minutes

Ingredients
- 2 tablespoons olive oil
- 2 red onions, chopped
- 1 green chilli, chopped
- 1 small tomato, chopped
- 3 eggs
- 1 teaspoon lemon juice
- ½ teaspoon turmeric powder
- ½ teaspoon red chilli powder
- 2 tablespoons coriander, chopped
- Salt to taste

Directions

In a bowl, combine chilli, coriander, green chillies, chopped onions and turmeric powder until well blended; whisk in the eggs and season with salt and pepper.

In a skillet, heat oil and then pour in about a third of the mixture; swirl the pan to spread the egg mixture and cook for about 1 minute per side or until the egg is set. Transfer to a plate and keep warm. Repeat with the remaining mixture. Serve hot with chilli sauce and a glass of fresh orange juice or chai for a satisfying breakfast meal.

Nutritional Info per Serving:

Calories: 241; Total Fat: 20.4 g; Carbs: 6.2 g; Dietary Fiber: 1.6 g; Sugars: 3.3 g; Protein: 9.2 g; Cholesterol: 246 mg; Sodium: 174 mg

6. Antioxidant-Rich Coconut & Blackberry Smoothie Bowl

Yield: 4 Servings
Total Time: 5 Minutes
Prep Time: 5 Minutes
Cook Time: N/A

Ingredients

- 2 cups fresh blackberries
- 2 cups fresh spinach
- 1 cup coconut milk
- 1 ripe avocado
- 2 tablespoons raw pumpkin seeds
- 2 tablespoons chia seeds
- ½ cup coconut flakes, toasted

Directions

In a blender, blend together almond milk, avocado, and spinach until very smooth and creamy; add in blackberries and pulse to combine well.
Divide the smooth among serving bowls and top each serving with fresh blackberries, pumpkin seeds, chia seeds and toasted coconut flakes.
Enjoy!

Nutritional Information per Serving:

Calories: 272; Total Fat: 20.7 g; Carbs: 15.2 g; Dietary Fiber: 9.6 g; Sugars: 9.8 g; Protein: 4.8 g; Cholesterol: 0 mg; Sodium: 25 mg

7. Spiced White Fish Breakfast Frittata

Yield: 2 Servings
Total Time: 30 Minutes
Prep Time: 10 Minutes
Cook Time: 20 Minutes

Ingredients:

- 1/2 cup white fish fillet, diced
- 1 tablespoon coconut oil
- 1 red onion, chopped
- 1 green pepper, chopped
- 2 garlic cloves, minced
- 1 ½ cups cherry tomatoes
- ½ teaspoon turmeric powder
- ½ teaspoon ground ginger
- ½ teaspoon cayenne pepper
- 1/2 teaspoon paprika
- 1 teaspoon cumin
- 6 free-range eggs beaten
- Pinch of sea salt
- Pinch of pepper
- 2 tablespoons chopped cilantro

Directions:

Preheat oven to 350°F. Melt coconut oil in oven-safe skillet and sauté red onion and green pepper; stir in garlic and cook for about 2 minutes or until fragrant. Stir in paprika, cayenne pepper, cumin, turmeric, ginger, salt and pepper and cook for about 1 minute; stir in tomatoes and cook until soft. Add in the fish and cover with eggs; season with salt and pepper and bake for about 15 minutes or until eggs are set. Serve warm garnished with cilantro.

Nutritional Information per Serving:

Calories: 344; Total Fat: 22 g; Carbs: 16 g; Dietary Fiber: 4.2 g; Sugars: 8.4 g; Protein: 23.5 g; Cholesterol: 500 mg; Sodium: 325 mg

8. Anti-Inflammatory Ginger Almond Blueberry Smoothie Bowl

Yield: 2 Servings
Total Time: 10 Minutes
Prep Time: 10 Minutes
Cook Time: N/A

Ingredients

- 1 cup unsweetened almond milk
- 1 scoop vanilla protein powder
- 1 tablespoon ground flaxseed
- 1 tablespoon almond butter
- 1 teaspoon minced fresh ginger
- 1 cup frozen, chopped spinach
- 1/4 cup frozen blueberries
- 2 tablespoons coconut flakes
- Extra blueberries for serving

Directions

Combine all ingredients in a blender and blend until very smooth and creamy. Divide the smoothie between serving bowls and top each with more blueberries and coconut flakes. Enjoy!

Nutrition information per Serving:

Calories: 222; Total Fat: 11.2 g; Carbs: 8.1 g; Dietary Fiber: 3.6 g; Sugars: 2.6 g; Protein: 3.7 g; Cholesterol: 0 mg; Sodium: 105 mg

9. Pan-Fried Mushrooms, Boiled Eggs, Spinach & Capsicum

Yield: 2 Servings
Total Time: 15 Minutes
Prep Time: 5 Minutes
Cook Time: 10 Minutes

Ingredients

- 4 large boiled eggs, diced
- 2 teaspoons extra-virgin olive oil
- 1/2 cup chopped button mushrooms
- 1 cup arugula/baby spinach
- 1/4 cup chopped red onion
- 1/4 cup chopped green bell pepper
- Hot sauce, to serve

Directions

Heat olive oil in a pan set over medium heat; add green bell pepper, onion and mushrooms and sauté for about 5 minutes or until tender.

Stir in arugula and cook for about 5 minutes or until it wilts; add diced boiled eggs and cook for a few minutes.

Serve right away with hot sauce.

Nutrition Information per Serving:

Calories: 201; Total Fat: 14.8 g; Carbs: 4.4 g; Dietary Fiber: 1 g; Sugars: 2.5 g Protein: 13.9 g; Cholesterol: 372 mg; Sodium: 216 mg

10. Healthy Keto Almond Flour Porridge

Yield: 2 Servings
Total Time: 7 Minutes
Prep Time: 2 Minutes
Cook Time: 5 Minutes

Ingredients

- 1 tablespoon ground flax
- ¼ cup Almond-Flour
- 3/4 cup water
- pinch of salt
- 1 large beaten egg
- 1/4 cup coconut milk
- 1 teaspoon stevia
- ½ cup fresh blackberries
- ¼ cup toasted chopped almonds

Directions

In a small pot set over medium-high heat, combine flax, almond flour, water and salt; lower heat and simmer for about 5 minutes, whisking constantly until the mixture thickens. Remove the pot from heat and gradually whisk in beaten egg until well combined. Return to heat and whisk until the porridge thickens. Remove from heat and continue whisking for about 30 seconds and then whisk in coconut milk and stevia. Serve garnished with berries and almonds.

Nutritional Information per Serving

Calories: 209; Total Fat: 16.7 g; Carbs: 9.2 g; Dietary fiber: 4.1 g; Sugars: 4.7 g; Protein: 9.5 g; Cholesterol: 98 mg; Sodium: 130 mg

11. Ground Beef, Eggs and Avocado Breakfast Bowl

Yield: 1 Serving
Total Time: 20 Minutes
Prep Time: 10 Minutes
Cook Time: 10 Minutes

Ingredients
- 2 eggs, lightly beaten
- 150g ground beef
- 8 medium mushrooms, sliced
- 1 red onion, sliced
- ½ tsp smoked paprika
- Salt & pepper
- 12 pitted black olives, sliced
- 1 small avocado, diced

Directions

Melt coconut oil in a skillet set over medium high heat; stir in mushrooms, onion, salt and pepper and cook for about 3 minutes or until veggies are tender and fragrant.
Stir in smoked paprika and ground beef; cook until beef is no longer pink; transfer to a plate. Add the eggs to the skillet and scramble for a few minutes; add in the beef mixture, olives and avocado and cook for about 1 minute. Transfer to a bowl and serve garnished with parsley.

Nutritional Information per Serving

Calories: 559; Total Fat: 47.5 g; Carbs: 2.6 g; Dietary fiber: 0.2 g; Sugars: 0.9 g; Protein: 30.4 g; Cholesterol: 445 mg; Sodium: 1132 mg

12. Low Carb Smoked Salmon Omelet

Yield: 1 Servings
Total Time: 20 Minutes
Prep Time: 10 Minutes
Cook Time: 10 Minutes

Ingredients

- 1 tsp. extra virgin olive oil
- 100 g sliced smoked salmon
- 1/2 tsp. capers
- 2 large eggs
- 10g chopped rocket
- 1 tsp. chopped parsley

Directions

Beat the eggs into a large bowl; stir in salmon, rocket, capers, and chopped parsley.
Add extra virgin olive oil to a nonstick pan and heat over medium heat until hot, but not
smoking; add the egg mixture and spread the mixture evenly in the pan. Lower heat and
cook until the omelet is cooked through.
With a spatula, roll up the omelet in half and serve hot.

Nutritional Information per Serving

*Calories: 303; Total Fat: 19 g; Carbs: 1.3 g; Dietary fiber: trace; Sugars: 1 g; Protein: 31.2 g;
Cholesterol: 395 mg; Sodium: 2186 mg*

13. Healthy Detox Porridge

Yield: 2 Servings
Total Time: 7 Minutes
Prep Time: 5 Minutes
Cook Time: 2 Minutes

Ingredients

- 1 cup unsweetened almond milk
- 2 tablespoons ground golden flax
- 1/2 cup coconut flour
- 1 tablespoon coconut oil
- 1 teaspoon cinnamon
- ¼ teaspoon salt
- 1 cup water
- 1 teaspoon stevia
- Toasted coconut to serve
- Toasted almonds to serve

Directions

In a microwave safe bowl, stir together all the ingredients until well combined; place in the microwave and heat for 1 minute. Stir again to mix well and microwave for another 1 minute. Serve right away topped with toasted almonds and toasted coconut.

Nutritional Information per Serving:

Calories: 267; Total Fat: 13.5 g; Carbs: 19.4 g; Dietary Fiber: 14.7 g; Sugars: 8.7 g; Protein: 5.9 g; Cholesterol: 0 mg; Sodium: 342 mg

14. Healthy Avocado Shrimp Omelet

Yields: 2 Servings
Total Time: 40 Minutes
Prep Time: 10 Minutes
Cook Time: 30 Minutes

Ingredients
- 1/4 pound shrimp, peeled and de-veined
- 4 large free-range eggs, beaten
- 1/2 medium avocado, diced
- 1 medium tomato, diced
- 1 teaspoon coconut oil
- 1/8 teaspoon freshly ground black pepper
- 1/4 teaspoon sea salt
- 1 tablespoon freshly chopped cilantro

Directions

Cook shrimp in a skillet set over medium heat until it turns pink; chop the cooked shrimp and set aside.

In a small bowl, toss together avocado, tomato, and cilantro; season with sea salt and pepper and set aside.

In a separate bowl, beat the eggs and set aside.

Set a skillet over medium heat; add coconut oil and heat until hot.

Add half of the egg to the skillet and tilt the skillet to cover the bottom. When almost cooked, add shrimp onto one side of the egg and fold in half. Cook for 1 minute more and top with the avocado-tomato mixture.

Repeat with the remaining ingredients for the second omelet.

Nutritional Information per Serving:

Calories: 344; Total Fat: 23.1 g; Carbs: 8.4 g; Dietary Fiber: 4.2 g; Protein: 27 g; Cholesterol: 491 mg; Sodium: 519 mg

15. Avocado and Egg Breakfast

Yield: 1 Serving
Total Time: 10 Minutes
Prep Time: 10 Minutes
Cook Time: N/A

Ingredients

- 1/2 avocado, diced
- 2 hard-boiled eggs
- Dash of hot sauce
- 1 teaspoon fresh herbs

Directions

Peel the boiled eggs and rinse with cold water; slice into four pieces each and add to a serving bowl. Add in diced avocado and serve garnished with fresh herbs and drizzled with hot sauce. Enjoy!

Nutritional Information per Serving:

Calories: 333; Total Fat: 28.4 g; Carbs: 9.8 g; Dietary Fiber: 7 g; Sugars: 1.2 g; Protein: 13.1 g; Cholesterol: 325 mg; Sodium: 145 mg

16. Low Carb Coconut Flour Pancakes

Total Time: 15 Minutes
Prep Time: 5 Minutes
Cook Time: 10 Minutes

Ingredients:
- 1/2 cup almond milk, unsweetened
- 1/2 cup coconut cream
- 1/2 cup coconut flour
- 2 tablespoons coconut oil, melted
- 4 free-range eggs
- 1/2 teaspoon baking soda
- 1/4 teaspoon Himalayan salt
- 1/2 teaspoon cinnamon
- 1 teaspoon vanilla
- Coconut oil for cooking

Directions

Combine all ingredients in a blender and blend until very smooth.
Heat coconut oil in a skillet set over medium heat; add in two spoonfuls of batter and spread into a circle. Cook for about 2 minutes per side or until browned.
Serve topped with fresh berries.

Nutritional Information per Serving:

Calories: 244 Total Fat: 23 g; Carbs: 4.9 g; Dietary Fiber: 2.7 g; Sugars: 1.5 g; Protein: 5.5 g; Cholesterol: 123 mg; Sodium: 296 mg

17. Healthy Scallions & Smoked Salmon Frittata

Yield: 6 servings
Total Time: 30 Minutes
Prep Time: 10 Minutes
Cook Time: 20 Minutes

Ingredients

- 2 teaspoons extra-virgin olive oil
- 6 scallions, trimmed and chopped
- 4 large eggs
- 6 large egg whites
- ½ teaspoon finely chopped fresh tarragon
- ¼ cup water
- ½ teaspoon salt
- 2 ounces smoked salmon, sliced into small pieces
- 2 tablespoons black olive tapenade

Directions

Preheat your oven to 350°F.

Set a large ovenproof pan over medium heat; add oil and heat until hot, but not smoky. Stir in scallions and sauté, stirring, for about 3 minutes or until tender and fragrant.

In a bowl, beat together eggs, egg whites, tarragon, water, and salt; season with black pepper and pour into the pan. Arrange the salmon onto the egg mixture. Cook, stirring frequently, for about 2 minutes or until almost set; transfer to the oven and cook for about 14 minutes or until puffed and golden. Remove the frittata from the oven and transfer to a serving plate; slice and serve with tapenade.

Nutritional Information per Serving:

Calories: 186; Total Fat: 5 g; Carbs: 1 g; Dietary Fiber: trace; Protein: 10 g; Cholesterol: 143 mg; Sodium: 535 mg; Sugars: trace

18. Spiced Egg Frittata

Yield: 4 Servings
Total Time: 20 Minutes
Prep Time: 10 Minutes
Cook Time: 10 Minutes

Ingredients

- 5 eggs
- 1 teaspoon paprika
- 1 tablespoon curry powder
- ½ teaspoon salt
- ½ teaspoon pepper
- 1 tablespoon chopped cilantro
- 1 cup diced tomatoes
- 2 tablespoons coconut oil
- 1 Serrano pepper, minced
- 1 yellow onion, diced

Directions

Preheat your oven to 350 degrees.

Whisk together eggs, spices and cilantro in a bowl; set aside.

Heat oil in a skillet and then fry in serrano peppers, onions, and salt until onion is soft; add in tomatoes and cook, covered, for 10 minutes or until tomatoes are soft. Add in the egg mixture and stir in to combine. Cook for about 5 minutes and then transfer to the oven. Bake for about minutes or until the egg is set. Serve hot with chai masala.

Nutritional Info per Serving:

Calories: 164; Total Fat: 1.9 g; Carbs: 6.3 g; Dietary Fiber: 2 g; Sugars: 3 g; Protein: 7.9 g; Cholesterol: 205 mg; Sodium: 373 mg

19. Omelets with Greens & Mushrooms

Yield: 2 Servings
Total Time: 25 Minutes
Prep Time: 10 Minutes
Cook Time: 15 Minutes

Ingredients

- 3 egg whites
- 1 egg
- 1/2 teaspoon extra-virgin olive oil
- 1/8 teaspoon red pepper flakes
- 1/8 teaspoon ground nutmeg
- 1/8 teaspoon garlic powder
- 1/4 teaspoon salt
- 1/8 teaspoon ground black pepper
- 1/2 cup sliced fresh mushrooms
- 2 tablespoons chopped red bell pepper
- 1/4 cup chopped green onion
- 1/2 cup chopped tomato
- 1 cup chopped fresh spinach

Directions

In a large bowl, whisk together egg whites, egg, garlic powder, red pepper flakes, nutmeg, salt and pepper until well blended.

Heat olive oil in a skillet over medium heat; add green onion, mushrooms and belle pepper and cook for about 5 minutes or until tender; stir in tomato and egg mixture and cook for about 5 minutes per side or until egg is set. Slice and serve hot.

Nutrition information per Serving:

Calories: 127; Total Fat: 4 g; Carbs: 13.7 g; Dietary Fiber: 3.1 g; Sugars: 8.4 g; Protein: 11 g; Cholesterol: 82 mg; Sodium: 392 mg

20. Immune Booster Breakfast Muesli

Yield: 1 Serving
Total Time: 10 Minutes + Chilling Time
Prep Time: 10 Minutes
Cook Time: N/A

Ingredients
- 1/2 cup fresh orange juice
- 1 cup gluten-free muesli
- 1/2 teaspoon raw honey
- 1/4 cup fresh elderberries
- 2 tablespoons blueberries
- 1/2 papaya, grated
- 1/4 cup Greek yoghurt
- 1 tablespoon chopped toasted cashew nuts
- 1 tablespoon toasted sesame seeds
- 1 tablespoon toasted pumpkin seeds

Directions

In a bowl, stir together fresh orange juice and muesli until well combined; refrigerate, covered, overnight. When ready, stir in raw honey, elderberries, blueberries, papaya, and Greek yogurt. Serve in a bowl and top with toasted nuts and seeds. Enjoy!

Nutritional Information Per Serving:

Calories: 251; Total Fat: 12.2; Carbs: 19.8 g; Dietary Fiber: 8.8 g; Sugars: 12.7; Protein: 14.2 g; Cholesterol: 10 mg; Sodium: 97 mg

21. Spiced Breakfast Egg Scramble

Yield: 1 Serving
Total Time: 20 Minutes
Prep Time: 10 Minutes
Cook Time: 10 Minutes

Ingredients

- 1 teaspoon coconut oil
- 1/8 red onion, diced
- 1/8 Bell Pepper, diced
- 1 teaspoon hot sauce
- 2 free-range eggs
- 1/4 teaspoon red pepper flakes, crushed
- 1/4 teaspoon cumin
- Pinch of sea salt
- Pinch of pepper

Directions

Melt coconut oil in a nonstick skillet set over medium heat; stir in red onions and peppers and sauté for about 4 minutes or until onions are translucent.

Meanwhile, in a bowl, whisk together hot sauce, eggs, crushed red pepper flakes, cumin, salt and pepper until frothy; add to onion mixture and cook, stirring, until eggs are set. Season with salt and pepper and serve with mango chutney.

Nutrition Information per Serving:

Calories: 203; Total Fat: 15.9 g; Carbs: 4.7 g; Dietary Fiber: 1 g; Sugars: 2.7 g Protein: 11.8 g; Cholesterol: 327 mg; Sodium: 528 mg

22. Low Carb Berry Shake

Yield: 4 Servings
Total Time: 5 Minutes
Prep Time: 5 Minutes
Cook Time: N/A

Ingredients
- ½ cup blackberries
- ½ cup strawberries
- ½ cup raspberries
- 2 cups coconut milk
- 1/4 cup peanut butter
- 1 teaspoon cinnamon
- 1 teaspoon liquid stevia
- 2 tablespoons almond butter

Directions

Blend everything together until very smooth. Enjoy!

Nutritional Information per Serving:

Calories: 378; Total Fat: 35.8 g; Carbs: 5.9 g; Dietary Fiber: 7 g; Sugars: 7.8 g; Protein: 5.3 g; Cholesterol: 0 mg; Sodium: 20 mg

23. Grain-Free Dairy-Free Pancakes

Yield: 4 Servings
Total Time: 26 Minutes
Prep Time: 10 Minutes
Cook Time: 16 Minutes

Ingredients

- 1 1/2 tablespoons coconut oil
- 3/4 cup coconut milk
- 8 eggs
- 1/4 cup tapioca flour
- 1/4 cup almond flour
- 100g whey protein powder
- 1 teaspoon salt
- ½ teaspoon chili powder
- ¼ teaspoon turmeric powder
- ¼ teaspoon black pepper
- ½ inch ginger, grated
- 1 serrano pepper, minced
- 1 handful cilantro, chopped
- ½ red onion, chopped

Directions

In a bowl, whisk eggs, coconut milk, tapioca flour, almond flour, protein powder, and spices until well blended; stir in ginger, Serrano pepper, cilantro, and red onion until well combined.

Melt coconut oil in a saucepan over medium low heat; add about ¼ cup of batter and spread out on the pan.
Cook for about 4 minutes per side or until golden brown.
Transfer to a plate and keep warm; repeat with the remaining batter and oil.
Serve the pancakes with freshly squeezed orange juice.

Nutritional Information per Serving:

Calories: 471; Total Fat: 31.2 g; Carbs: 23.9 g; Dietary Fiber: 3.1g; Sugars: 4.2 g; Protein: 26.9 g; Cholesterol: 330 mg; Sodium: 787 mg

24. Curried Egg Frittata

Yield: 4 Servings
Total Time: 20 Minutes
Prep Time: 10 Minutes
Cook Time: 10 Minutes

Ingredients

- 5 eggs
- 1 teaspoon paprika
- 1 tablespoon curry powder
- ½ teaspoon salt
- ½ teaspoon pepper
- 1 tablespoon chopped cilantro
- 1 cup diced tomatoes
- 2 tablespoons coconut oil
- 1 Serrano pepper, minced
- 1 yellow onion, diced

Directions

Preheat your oven to 350 degrees.
Whisk together eggs, spices and cilantro in a bowl; set aside.
Heat oil in a skillet and then fry in serrano peppers, onions, and salt until onion is soft; add in tomatoes and cook, covered, for 10 minutes or until tomatoes are soft. Add in the egg mixture and stir in to combine. Cook for about 5 minutes and then transfer to the oven. Bake for about minutes or until the egg is set. Serve hot with chai masala.

Nutritional Info per Serving:

Calories: 164; Total Fat: 1.9 g; Carbs: 6.3 g; Dietary Fiber: 2 g; Sugars: 3 g; Protein: 7.9 g; Cholesterol: 205 mg; Sodium: 373 mg

25. Healthy Lunch Salad with Hot Creamy Avocado Dressing

Yield: 4 Servings
Total Time: 5 Minutes
Prep Time: 5 Minutes
Cook Time: N/A

Ingredients

Salad
- ¼ cup blueberries
- ½ cup chopped strawberries
- 1 cup chopped kale
- 1 cup arugula
- 1 cup baby spinach
- 2 chopped red onions
- 1 cup shredded carrots
- 1 cup diced tomatoes

Hot Creamy Dressing
- 1 tablespoon extra-virgin olive oil
- 1/4 cup fresh lemon juice
- ¼ cup fresh orange juice
- 1/2 cup fresh elderberries
- 1 avocado
- 1 tablespoon raw honey
- 1 teaspoon sea salt
- ½ teaspoon cayenne pepper

Directions
In a blender, blend together all dressing ingredients until very smooth and creamy; set aside.
Combine all salad ingredients in a large bowl; drizzle with dressing and toss to coat well before serving.

Nutritional Information per Serving:

Calories: 141; Total Fat: 7.4 g; Carbs: 17.4 g; Dietary Fiber: 5.5 g; Sugars: 7.5 g; Protein: 2.9 g; Cholesterol: 0 mg; Sodium: 42 mg

26. Scrumptious Beef & Green Bean Stir-Fry

Yield: 4 Servings
Total Time: 20 Minutes
Prep Time: 5 Minutes
Cook Time: 15 Minutes

Ingredients
- 500g lean beef mince
- 2 cups sliced green beans
- 1 cup freshly squeezed pineapple juice
- 1 tablespoon oyster sauce
- 2 long fresh red chillies, sliced
- 1/3 cup chopped mint leaves
- 1 cup fresh coriander sprigs
- 3 garlic cloves, sliced
- Steamed brown rice

Directions

Heat oil in a skillet set over medium heat; sauté garlic for about 2 minutes or until fragrant; transfer to a plate and add beef to the skillet. Fry for about 5 minutes or until browned. Add in seasoning and cook for one minute; stir in pineapple juice and oyster sauce. Simmer for about 10 minutes or until the mixture in thick.

Stir in beans and cook for about 2 minutes or until crisp. Stir in mint and coriander and serve sprinkled with garlic and chilli. Serve over hot brown rice.

Nutritional Information per Serving:
Calories: 274; Total Fat: 4.1 g; Carbs: 16 g; Dietary Fiber: 5 g; Sugars: 6 g; Protein: 32 g; Cholesterol: 82 mg; Sodium: 213 mg

27. Barbecued Steak Salad with Thai Dressing

Yield: 4 Servings
Total Time: 30 Minutes
Prep Time: 20 Minutes
Cook Time: 10 Minutes

Ingredients
- 500g lean beef steaks
- 1 cup green salad
- 2 heads baby lettuce
- 2 radishes, sliced
- 1 nectarine, pitted and sliced
- 1 carrot, peeled, shaved
- 3 baby cucumbers, shaved
- 1 cup fresh coriander leaves
- 1 cup small fresh mint leaves

Thai Dressing
- 4 tablespoons olive oil, divided
- 1/4 cup fresh lime juice
- 1 red bird's eye chilli, chopped
- 1 tablespoon grated peeled ginger
- 2 tablespoons chopped shallot
- 2 tablespoons fish sauce

Directions

Preheat your BBQ grill on medium high.
In a blender, blend together shallot, fish sauce, three tablespoons of olive oil, lime juice, chilli, ginger and raw honey until very smooth; set aside.
Brush the remaining oil over the steaks and sprinkle with salt and pepper; barbecue the meat for about 4 minutes per side or until cooked through.
Transfer the steak to a chopping board and slice into small pieces.
Divide salad mix, lettuce leaves, radishes, cucumbers, nectarine, carrots, coriander, and mint on serving plates and drizzle with the Thai dressing; toss to coat well. Top each serving with sliced steak and serve with the remaining dressing. Enjoy!

Nutritional Information per Serving:

Calories: 385; Total Fat: 23 g; Carbs: 11 g; Dietary Fiber: 8 g; Sugars: 3 g; Protein: 30 g; Cholesterol: 112 mg; Sodium: 1132 mg

28. Stir-Fried Mushrooms & Spinach with Golden Onions

Yield: 6 Servings
Total Time: 35 Minutes
Prep Time: 15 Minutes
Cook Time: 20 Minutes

Ingredients

- 1 cup chestnut mushrooms, quartered
- 2 medium onions, chop one and thinly slice the other
- 6 cups ready washed young leaf spinach
- 3 tablespoons sunflower oil
- 1 small green chilli, chopped
- 1 tablespoon minced ginger
- 1 crushed garlic clove
- ½ teaspoon garlic
- ½ teaspoon garam masala
- ½ teaspoon cumin seeds
- ½ teaspoon turmeric

Directions

Heat two tablespoons of oil in a large pan; fry in cumin seeds for 30 seconds or until fragrant and then add in onion and mushrooms; cook for 10 minutes or until tender. Stir in chilli, ginger, garlic and garam masala. Stir in spinach and cook for 3 minutes or until wilted. Season with salt and serve warm.

In the remaining oil, fry onion slices with turmeric for about 7 minutes or until golden browned. Serve the spinach sprinkled with onions.

Nutritional Information per Serving:

Calories: 103; Total Fat: 7 g; Carbs: 5 g; Dietary Fiber: 4 g; Sugars: 0 g; Protein: 5 g; Cholesterol: 11 mg; Sodium: 510 mg

29. Spicy cauliflower

Yield: 8 Servings
Total Time: 30 Minutes
Prep Time: 10 Minutes
Cook Time: 20 Minutes

Ingredients

- 1¼kg cauliflower, broken into pieces
- 1 tablespoon chopped ginger
- 6 tablespoons vegetable oil
- 2 teaspoon turmeric
- 2 tablespoons cumin seed
- 2 teaspoons chilli flakes
- 1 tablespoon chopped coriander

Directions

Heat oil in a wok and stir in ginger and all the spices for about 40 seconds or until fragrant; lower heat and stir in cauliflower and seasoning. Cook, covered, for 10 minutes or until tender and then remove from heat. Serve garnished with coriander.

Nutritional Information per Serving:

Calories: 145; Total Fat: 10 g; Carbs: 7 g; Dietary Fiber: 3 g; Sugars: 4 g; Protein: 6 g; Cholesterol: 3 mg; Sodium: 50 mg

30. Charred Chicken with Healthy Broccoli Salad

Yield: 4 Servings
Total Time: 35 Minutes
Prep Time: 15 Minutes
Cook Time: 20 Minutes

Ingredients

- 4 large skinless chicken thigh cutlets
- 1 1/2 tablespoons gluten-free Cajun seasoning
- 1/4 cup extra virgin olive oil
- 300g broccoli, grated
- 1 carrot, coarsely grated
- 1/2 small red onion, thinly sliced
- 1/4 cup lemon juice
- 1 tablespoon drained baby capers
- 1 lemon, cut into wedges, to serve

Directions

Drizzle chicken with oil and sprinkle with seasoning; rub to coat well.

Preheat your grill on medium heat; cook chicken for about 15 minutes, turning severally, until cooked through.

In the meantime, place the grated broccoli in a bowl and add in red onion, carrots, capers, lime juice and the remaining oil, salt and pepper; toss to combine well and serve with grilled chicken garnished with lemon wedges.

Nutritional Information per Serving:

Calories: 425; Total Fat: 26 g; Carbs: 9.5 g; Dietary Fiber: 6.2 g; Sugars: 2.3 g; Protein: 40.3 g; Cholesterol: 154 mg; Sodium: 396 mg

Yield: 4 Servings
Total Time: 15 Minutes
Prep Time: 15 Minutes
Cook Time: N/A

Ingredients
- 4 (100g) skin-on mackerel fillets
- 1/8 teaspoon sea salt
- 2 teaspoons extra virgin olive oil
- 4 cups arugula
- 8 leaves Boston lettuce, washed and dried
- 1 cup snow peas, cooked
- 2 avocados, diced

For Grapefruit-Dill Dressing:
- 1/4 cup grapefruit juice
- 1/4 cup extra virgin olive oil
- 1 teaspoon raw honey
- 1 tablespoon Dijon mustard
- 1 tablespoon chopped fresh dill
- 2 garlic cloves, minced
- 1/2 teaspoon salt

Directions

Sprinkle fish with about 1/8 teaspoon salt and cook in 2 teaspoons of olive oil over medium heat for about 4 minutes per side or until golden.

In a small bowl, whisk together al dressing ingredients and set aside.

Divide arugula and lettuce among four serving plates

Divide lettuce and arugula among 4 plates and add the remaining salad ingredients; top each with seared fish and drizzle with dressing. Enjoy!

Nutritional Information per Serving:

Calories: 608; Total Fat: 46 g; Carbs: 16.2 g; Dietary Fiber: 8.7 g; Sugars: 5.1 g; Protein: 38.9 g; Cholesterol: 78 mg; Sodium: 488 mg

32. Steamed Chicken with Mushroom and Ginger

Yield: 4 Servings
Total Time: 20 Minutes
Prep Time: 10 Minutes
Cook Time: 10 Minutes

Ingredients
- 4 x 150g chicken breast fillets
- 2 teaspoons extra-virgin olive oil
- 1 1/2 tablespoons balsamic vinegar
- 8cm piece ginger, cut into matchsticks
- 1 bunch broccoli
- 1 bunch carrots, diced
- 6 small dried shiitake mushrooms, chopped
- Spring onion, sliced
- Fresh coriander leaves,

Directions

In a bowl, combine sliced chicken with salt, vinegar, and pepper; let marinate for at least 10 minutes.

Transfer the chicken to a baking dish and scatter with mushrooms and ginger; cook in a preheated oven at 350 degrees for about 15 minutes; place chopped broccoli and carrots on top of the chicken and return to the oven. Cook for another 3 minutes or until chicken is tender.

Divide the chicken, broccoli, and carrots on serving plates and drizzle each with olive oil and top with coriander and red onions. Enjoy!

Nutritional Information per Serving:

Calories: 242; Total Fat: 5 g; Carbs: 10 g; Dietary Fiber: 4 g; Sugars: 2 g; Protein: 37 g; Cholesterol: 88 mg; Sodium: 114 mg

Yield: 2 Servings
Total Time: 10 Minutes
Prep Time: 10 Minutes

Ingredients

For the Salad
- 2 (150g each) pre-grilled white fish
- ½ cup snap peas, sliced
- 1 cup baby spinach
- 1 cup chopped Romaine lettuce
- ½ cup avocado, sliced
- ½ cup blueberries
- 2 green onions, sliced
- ½ cup shredded carrot
- 1 large cucumber, chopped
- 1 tablespoon chia seeds

For the Dressing
- 1 clove garlic, minced
- ¼ teaspoon oregano
- 1 tablespoon tahini
- 1 teaspoon honey
- 1 tablespoon rice wine vinegar
- 1 tablespoon lemon juice
- 1 teaspoon sesame oil
- 1/8 teaspoon red pepper flakes
- ¼ teaspoon salt
- ¼ teaspoon black pepper

Directions

In a large bowl, combine all salad ingredients, except fish.
In a small bowl, whisk together all dressing ingredients until well blended; pour over the salad and toss until well blended. Top each serving with the grilled white fish and enjoy!

Nutritional Information per Serving:

Calories: 256; Total Fat: 14.1 g; Carbs: 29.7 g; Dietary Fiber: 8.5 g; Sugars: 13.5 g; Protein: 6.5 g; Cholesterol: 0 mg; Sodium: 343 mg

Yield: 6 Servings
Total Time: 10 Minutes
Prep Time: 10 Minutes
Cook Time: N/A

Ingredients

For the salad:
- 1 kg lean steak
- ¼ cup freshly squeezed lime juice
- A pinch of sea salt
- A pinch of pepper
- 2 large carrots, grated
- 1 red bell pepper, cut into matchsticks
- 2 cups broccoli florets
- 2 cups thinly sliced red cabbage
- 2 cups kale, thinly sliced
- 1 cup walnuts
- 2 avocados, diced
- 1/2 cup chopped parsley
- 1 tablespoon sesame seeds

For the dressing:
- 1/2 cup lemon juice, fresh
- 1/3 cup grape seed oil
- 2 teaspoons whole grain mustard
- 1 tablespoon grated fresh ginger
- 1/4 teaspoon sea salt
- 1 teaspoon raw honey

Directions

In a small dish, mix lime juice, salt and pepper; spread over the steak and grill on a preheated charcoal grill for about 8 minutes per side or until cooked to your liking.
In a small bowl, whisk together all the dressing ingredients until well blended; set aside.

In a large bowl, combine carrots, bell pepper, broccoli, cabbage, and kale; pour over the dressing and toss until well coated. Add walnuts, avocado, and parsley and sesame seeds and toss to mix well. Top with the grilled steak and enjoy!

Nutritional Information per Serving:

Calories: 332; Total Fat: 26.6 g; Carbs: 20.2 g; Dietary Fiber: 9 g; Sugars: 5.5 g; Protein: 3.1 g; Cholesterol: 0 mg; Sodium: 138 mg

Yield: 4 Servings
Total Time: 20 Minutes
Prep Time: 10 Minutes
Cook Time: 10 Minutes

Ingredients

- 400g grilled lean steak
- 2 cups shiitake mushrooms
- 1 tablespoon balsamic vinegar
- 1/4 cup extra virgin olive oil
- 1-2 garlic cloves, minced
- A handful of parsley
- 1 teaspoon salt

Directions

Rinse the mushroom and pat dry; put in a foil and drizzle with balsamic vinegar and extra virgin olive oil.
Sprinkle the mushroom with garlic, parsley, and salt.
Grill for about 10 minutes or until tender and cooked through. Serve warm with grilled steak.

Nutritional Information per Serving:

Calories: 171; Total Fat: 12.8g; Carbs: 15.9g; Dietary Fiber: 2.4g; Protein: 1.8g; Cholesterol: 0mg; Sodium: 854mg; sugars: 4.1g

36.Clean Eating Lemon Grilled Salmon & Avocado Vegetable Salad

Yield: 3 Servings
Total Time: 10 Minutes
Prep Time: 10 Minutes
Cook Time: N/A

Ingredients

- 3 (150g each) salmon fillet
- ¼ cup freshly squeezed lemon juice
- A pinch of sea salt
- A pinch of pepper
- 1 small red onion, sliced into thin rings
- 1 cup watercress, rinsed
- 1 zucchini, shaved
- 1 small broccoli head, rinsed and cut in small florets
- 1 avocado, diced
- 2 tablespoon s fresh lemon juice
- 1 tablespoon extra-virgin olive oil
- ½ teaspoon Dijon mustard
- ½ teaspoon sea salt
- ¼ cup crushed toasted almonds
- 1 tablespoon chia seeds

Directions

In a bowl, mix lemon juice, salt and pepper until well combined; smear on the fish fillets until well coated and grill on a preheated charcoal grill for about 7 minutes per side or until browned and cooked to your liking.

In another bowl, mix together the veggies until well combined.

In a small bowl, whisk together lemon juice, olive oil, mustard and salt until well blended; pour over the salad and toss until well coated.

Add almonds and chia seeds and toss to combine. Set the salad aside for at least 5 minutes for flavors to combine before serving.

Serve the salad drizzled with the dressing and topped with the grilled salmon for a healthy satisfying meal.

Nutritional Information per Serving:

Calories: 258; Total Fat: 22.1 g; Carbs: 14.1 g; Dietary Fiber: 7.7 g; Sugars: 3.5 g; Protein: 5.3 g; Cholesterol: 0 mg; Sodium: 352 mg

37. Beef Stir Fry with Red Onions & Cabbage

Yield: 4 Servings
Total Time: 20 Minutes
Prep Time: 10 Minutes
Cook Time: 10 Minutes

Ingredients:

- 550g grass-fed flank steak, thinly sliced strips
- 1 tablespoon apple cider wine
- 2 teaspoons balsamic vinegar
- Pinch of sea salt
- pinch of pepper
- 4 tablespoons extra-virgin olive oil
- 1 large yellow onion, thinly chopped
- 1/2 red bell pepper, thinly sliced
- 1/2 green bell pepper, thinly sliced
- 1 tablespoon toasted sesame seeds
- 1 teaspoon crushed red pepper flakes
- 4 cups cabbage
- 1 ½ avocados, diced

Directions:

Place meat in a bowl; stir in rice wine and vinegar, sea salt and pepper. Toss to coat well. Heat a tablespoon of olive oil in a pan set over medium high heat; add meat and cook for about 2 minutes or until meat is browned; stir for another 2 minutes and then remove from heat. Heat the remaining oil to the pan and sauté onions for about 2 minutes or until caramelized; stir in pepper and cook for 2 minutes more. Stir in cabbage and cook for 2 minutes; return meat to pan and stir in sesame seeds and red pepper flakes. Serve hot topped with diced avocado!

Nutritional Info per Serving:

Calories: 459; Fat: 30 g; Carbs: 16.6 g; Dietary Fiber: 6.1 g; Sugars: 7.8 g; Protein: 35.3 g; Cholesterol: 112 mg; Sodium: 516 mg

38.Grilled Chicken with Rainbow Salad Bowl

Yield: 2 Servings
Total Time: 15 Minutes
Prep Time: 15 Minutes
Cook Time: N/A

Ingredients

- 300g grilled skinless chicken, shredded
- 2 cups mixed salad leaves
- 4 radishes, thinly sliced
- 1 cup chopped tomatoes
- 1 cup shredded carrot
- 1 cup podded edamame
- 4 tablespoons almond butter
- 2 tablespoons freshly squeezed lemon juice
- 2 tablespoons freshly squeezed lime juice
- ½ teaspoon sea salt

Directions

Blanch edamame in boiling water for about 2 minutes and then drain; transfer to a serving bowl and add in salad leaves, radish, tomatoes, carrots and chicken.
In a bowl, whisk together fresh lemon juice, lime juice, almond butter, and sea salt until smooth; drizzle over the salad and serve.

Nutritional Information per Serving:

Calories: 292; Total Fat: 9 g; Carbs: 19.6 g; Dietary Fiber: 12.3 g; Sugars: 6 g; Protein: 27.8 g; Cholesterol: 30 mg; Sodium: 330 mg

39.Turkey & Coconut Soup

Yield: 2 Servings
Total Time: 40 Minutes
Prep Time: 10 Minutes
Cook Time: 30 Minutes

Ingredients

- 1 tsp. coconut oil
- 1 red onion, finely sliced
- 1 ginger, finely chopped
- 1 clove garlic, finely chopped
- 1 lemon grass, bashed with a rolling pin
- 2 sticks celery, diced
- 1/4 cup coconut milk
- ½ cup vegetable stock
- 8 oz. turkey, cooked, roughly chopped
- 1/8 tsp. sea salt
- 1/8 tsp. black pepper
- 1 cup coriander, finely chopped
- 1 cup spinach, roughly chopped
- 2 tbsp. fresh lime juice

Directions

Add coconut oil to a medium pan set over medium heat; stir in red onions and sauté for about 5 minutes or until translucent. Add ginger and garlic and sauté for about 3 minutes or until garlic is golden.

Stir in lemon grass, celery, coconut milk, and vegetable sock; bring to a simmer. Simmer for about 15 minutes or until celery is soft.

Stir in turkey, salt and black pepper; cook for about 5 minutes or until turkey is cooked heated through.

Remove from heat and stir in coriander and spinach; serve into soup bowls and sprinkle with a squeeze of lime juice and coriander.

Nutritional Information per Serving:

Calories: 327; Total Fat: 15.4 g; Carbs: 11.2 g; Dietary Fiber: 3.4 g; Sugars: 4.4 g; Protein: 35.8 g; Cholesterol: 86 mg; Sodium: 276 mg

40.Pepper Beef and Lettuce Wraps

Yield: 8 Servings
Total Time: 30 Minutes
Prep Time: 25 Minutes
Cook Time: 5 Minutes

Ingredients

- 450g lean diced beef
- 1 tablespoon extra-virgin olive oil
- 1 teaspoon black pepper
- 1 teaspoon white pepper
- 1 teaspoon salt
- 1 cup bean sprouts, trimmed
- 16 baby cos lettuce leaves
- 1 large red onion, diced
- 12 fresh lemon wedges
- 16 large fresh mint leaves

Directions

Preheat your pan over medium high heat; in a bowl, mix together oil, white pepper, salt and black pepper until well combined; add in beef and toss to coat well. Grill for about 5 minutes per side or until cooked through. Let rest for at least 5 minutes.
Arrange lettuce leaves on serving plates and top each mint and bean sprouts. Serve topped with sliced beef and garnished with lemon wedges.

Nutritional Information per Serving:

Calories: 121; Total Fat: 4.1 g; Carbs: 7.2 g; Dietary Fiber: 1.9 g; Sugars: 6 g; Protein: 16.9 g; Cholesterol: 30 mg; Sodium: 330 mg

41.Low Carb Berry Salad with Citrus Dressing

Yield: 3 Servings
Total Time: 5 Minutes
Prep Time: 5 Minutes
Cook Time: N/A

Ingredients

Salad
- ¼ cup blueberries
- ½ cup chopped strawberries
- 1 cup mixed greens (kale and chard)
- 2 cups baby spinach
- 2 chopped green onions
- ½ cup chopped avocado
- 1 shredded carrots

Citrus Dressing
- 1 tablespoon extra-virgin olive oil
- 2 tablespoons apple cider vinegar
- ¼ cup fresh orange juice
- 5 strawberries chopped

Directions

In a blender, blend together all dressing ingredients until very smooth; set aside.
Combine all salad ingredients in a large bowl; drizzle with dressing and toss to coat well
before serving.

Nutritional Information per Serving:

*Calories: 141; Total Fat: 7.4 g; Carbs: 17.4 g; Dietary Fiber: 5.5 g; Sugars: 7.5 g; Protein: 2.9 g;
Cholesterol: 0 mg; Sodium: 42 mg*

Yield: 4 Servings
Total Time: 25 Minutes
Prep Time: 5 Minutes
Cook Time: 20 Minutes

Ingredients

- 4 cups cauliflower florets
- 8 cups broccoli florets
- 1 tablespoon extra-virgin olive oil
- 1 celery rib, chopped
- 1 small onion, chopped
- 1/8 teaspoon celery seeds
- 1/4 teaspoon white pepper
- 1/2 teaspoon onion powder
- 1/2 teaspoon garlic powder
- 1 teaspoon salt
- 3 cups vegetable broth
- 1 cup coconut milk

Directions

In a stock pot, heat olive oil over medium heat and then stir in celery, onion, salt and pepper; cook for about 3 minutes or until fragrant. Stir in celery seeds, garlic powder, onion powder, cauliflower, half of broccoli and vegetable broth. Simmer covered, for about 10 minutes. Transfer the mixture, in batches, to a blender and blend until very smooth; return to the pot. Chop the remaining broccoli and add to the pot along with coconut milk. Simmer for about 3 minutes and then remove from heat to serve.

Nutritional Information per Serving:

Calories: 151; Total Fat: 5 g; Carbs: 23 g; Dietary Fiber: 8 g; Sugars: 8g; Protein: 8.1 g; Cholesterol: 0 mg; Sodium: 1457 mg

43.Green Salad with Beets & Edamame

Yield: 2 Servings
Total Time: 15 Minutes
Prep Time: 15 Minutes
Cook Time: N/A

Ingredients

- ½ cup shredded raw beet
- 1 cup shelled edamame, thawed
- 2 cups mixed salad greens
- 2 teaspoons extra-virgin olive oil
- 1 tablespoon + 1½ teaspoons apple cider vinegar
- 1 tablespoon chopped fresh cilantro
- Salt & pepper

Directions

In a large bowl, combine beets, edamame and salad greens. In a small bowl, whisk together olive oil, vinegar, cilantro, salt and pepper and drizzle over the salad. Serve chilled.

Nutrition information per Serving:

Calories: 325; Total Fat: 16 g; Carbs: 25 g; Dietary Fiber: 12 g; Sugars: 6 g; Protein: 18 g; Cholesterol: 0 mg; Sodium: 499 mg;

Yields: 8 Servings
Total Time: 17 Minutes
Prep Time: 5 Minutes
Cook Time: 12 Minutes

Ingredients
- 2 pounds white fish, diced
- 1 tablespoon vegetable oil
- 1/4 cup tamarind juice
- 1/2 teaspoon cumin seeds
- 1 tablespoon ground turmeric
- 1 tablespoon red chile powder
- 1 1/2 teaspoons salt
- 2 tablespoons red chile powder
- 2 tablespoons ground coriander
- 1 1/2 tablespoons garlic paste
- 1 large onion, minced
- 1 tablespoon chopped coriander
- 1 cup warm water
- 1/4 cup oil
- 1 pinch salt

Directions

Add fish in a large bowl, and then add in turmeric, chile powder, oil, and salt; let marinate for at least 10 minutes.

Heat about 1/4 in a skillet set over medium heat; stir in cumin seeds and onions; sauté for about 10 minutes. Stir in garlic paste and cook for 3 minutes and then add in carp fish and cook for 5 minutes. Stir in tamarind juice and add in coriander, chile powder and salt. Cook for about 10 minutes or until the sauce is thick.

Serve garnished with coriander leaves.

Nutritional Info per Serving:

Calories: 180; Total Fat: 10.6 g; Carbs: 6.3 g; Dietary Fiber: 2.8 g; Sugars: 1.9 g; Protein: 14.2 g; Cholesterol: 50 mg; Sodium: 428 mg

45.Chicory & orange salad with ginger dressing

Yield: 8 Servings
Total Time: 10 Minutes
Prep Time: 10 Minutes
Cook Time: N/A

Ingredients

For the dressing
- 1/2 cup groundnut oil
- 2 teaspoons clear honey
- 3 tablespoons fresh lemon juice
- 2 tablespoons orange juice
- ½ teaspoon finely grated orange zest
- 1 teaspoon Dijon mustard
- 1 garlic clove, crushed
- 2 teaspoons freshly grated ginger

For the salad
- 85g bag watercress, large stalks removed and chopped
- 50g bag lamb's lettuce, chopped
- 2 large heads of chicory, chopped
- 3 oranges, peeled, segmented, and deseeded

Directions

In a jar, combine all dressing ingredients and shake to mix well. Chill in the refrigerator for at least 2 days before using.
Combine all salad ingredients and chill for at least 1 hour. When ready, drizzle with dressing and mix to coat well. Enjoy!

Nutritional Information per Serving:

Calories: 143; Total Fat: 12 g; Carbs: 8 g; Dietary Fiber: 2 g; Sugars: 1 g; Protein: 2 g; Cholesterol: 0 mg; Sodium: 70 mg

46. Anti-Inflammatory Spiced Carrot Soup

Yield: 4 Servings
Total Time: 50 Minutes
Prep Time: 10 Minutes
Cook Time: 40 Minutes

Ingredients

- 1 tablespoon olive oil
- 1 cup chopped leek
- 1 cup chopped butternut squash
- 1 cup chopped fennel
- 3 cups chopped carrots
- 1 tablespoon turmeric
- 1 tablespoon grated ginger
- 2 garlic cloves, minced
- 2 cups coconut milk
- 3 cups vegetable broth
- Salt & pepper

Directions

Heat oil in a saucepan and then sauté in leeks, fennel, squash, and carrots for about 5 minutes or until tender. Stir in turmeric, ginger, garlic, salt and pepper and cook for about 2 minutes. Stir in coconut milk and broth and simmer for about 20 minutes.
Transfer the mixture to a blender and blend until creamy. Serve right away with a dollop of yogurt.

Nutritional Information per Serving:

Calories: 210; Total Fat: 10.9 g; Carbs: 25.6 g; Dietary Fiber: 4.8 g; Sugars: 7.7g; Protein: 2.1 g; Cholesterol: 0 mg; Sodium: 875 mg

47.Healthy Salad with Grilled Chicken Wrap

Yield: 2 Servings
Total Time: 10 Minutes
Prep Time: 10 Minutes
Cook Time: N/A

Ingredients

- 2 lettuce leaves
- ½ coddled egg
- 1 cup diced cherry tomatoes
- 6 cups chopped curly kale
- 8 ounces sliced grilled chicken
- 1 clove garlic, minced
- 1/2 teaspoon Dijon mustard
- 1 teaspoon raw honey
- 1/8 cup olive oil
- 1/8 cup fresh lemon juice
- Salt & pepper

Directions

In a large bowl, whisk together half of the egg, honey, mustard, minced garlic, olive oil, fresh lemon juice, salt and pepper until well combined.
Add in cherry tomatoes, chicken and kale and toss to coat well; spread the mixture onto lettuce leaves and roll to form wraps. Slice in half and serve right away!

Nutritional Information per Serving:

Calories: 386; Total Fat: 16.9 g; Carbs: 28.5 g; Dietary Fiber: 4.3 g; Sugars: 5.7 g; Protein: 32.5 g; Cholesterol: 114 mg; Sodium: 183 mg

Yield: 4 Servings
Total Time: 25 Minutes
Prep Time: 10 Minutes
Cook Time: 15 Minutes

Ingredients

- 2 pounds medium shrimp, deveined
- 1/4 cup vegetable oil
- 1 large onion, chopped
- 1 teaspoon ground red chile pepper
- 1 tablespoon ginger garlic paste
- 1 tomato, finely chopped
- 1 teaspoon ground coriander
- 1/2 teaspoon ground turmeric
- 10 fresh curry leaves
- 1 teaspoon garam masala
- chopped fresh cilantro
- 1/4 cup water
- 2/3 teaspoon salt

Directions

Heat oil in a large saucepan and then sauté onions for about 5 minutes or until fragrant and lightly browned; stir in ginger, cilantro, curry leaves, garlic paste, and salt. Cook for 1 minute.

Mix in shrimp, tomato, turmeric, chile powder and water; lower heat and cook for 8 minutes or until shrimp is no longer pink. Season with garam masala and then remove from heat. Serve over rice or flat bread, garnished with cilantro. Enjoy!

Nutritional Information per Serving:

Calories: 270; Total Fat: 12.8 g; Carbs: 5.3 g; Dietary Fiber: 2.8 g; Sugars: 2.7 g; Protein: 30.7 g; Cholesterol: 277 mg; Sodium: 734 mg

49.Grilled Beef & Steamed Veggie Salad with Macadamia Dressing

Yield: 3 Servings
Total Time: 15 Minutes
Prep Time: 10 Minutes
Cook Time: 5 Minutes

Ingredients

For the Dressing
- 2 tablespoons freshly squeezed orange juice
- 2 tablespoons freshly squeezed lemon juice
- 3 tablespoons extra-virgin olive oil
- 1/2 teaspoon raw honey
- 1 teaspoon raw apple-cider vinegar
- 4 fresh sliced basil leaves
- 1 1/2 tablespoons chopped fresh parsley
- 1 1/2 tablespoons chopped fresh dill
- 1/4 cup toasted and chopped macadamia nuts
- ¼ teaspoon coarse salt

For the Salad
- 3/4 pound grilled beef
- 1 cup asparagus, trimmed
- 1/2 cup carrots, scrubbed
- 1/4 pound green beans, trimmed
- 1/2 large fennel bulb, cut into 1/2-inch slices
- ½ tsp. coarse salt

Directions

In a bowl, whisk together the dressing ingredients and season with salt; set aside.
Steam veggies in steamer set over a saucepan of boiling water for about 5 minutes or until crisp tender.
Half the steamed carrots and asparagus spears lengthwise.

Arrange the veggies on a serving platter and sprinkle with salt; drizzle with the dressing and garnish with herbs.

Macros Breakdown:

Calories: 515; Fat: 35.8 g; Carbs: 13.8 g; Dietary Fiber: 7.2 g; Sugars: 2.2 g; Protein: 39.3 g; Cholesterol: 255 mg; Sodium: 581 mg

50.Vegetable Detox Soup

Yield: 4 Servings
Total Time: 35 Minutes
Prep Time: 15 Minutes
Cook Time: 20 Minutes

Ingredients

- 1/4 cup water
- 2 cloves garlic, minced
- 1/2 of a red onion, diced
- 1 tablespoon fresh ginger, peeled and minced
- 1 small head of cauliflower, chopped
- 3 medium carrots, diced
- 3 celery stalks, diced
- 6 cups water
- 1/4 teaspoon cinnamon
- 1 teaspoon turmeric
- 1/8 teaspoon cayenne pepper
- Sea salt
- Freshly ground black pepper
- juice of 1 lemon
- 1 cup green cabbage, chopped
- 2 cups kale, torn in pieces

Directions

Bring a large pot of water to a gentle boil over medium heat. Add garlic and onion and cook for about 2 minutes, stirring occasionally. Stir in fresh ginger, cauliflower, carrots, and celery and continue cooking for 3 minutes more. Stir in cinnamon, turmeric, cayenne pepper, sea salt and black pepper.
Add in ½ cup water and bring the mixture to a rolling boil; reduce heat and simmer for about 15 minutes or until the veggies and tender. Stir in lemon juice, cabbage, and kale during the last 2 minutes of cooking. Serve hot or warm.

Nutritional Information per Serving

Calories: 74; Total Fat: 0.4 g; Carbs: 16.1 g; Dietary fiber: 4.1 g; Protein: 3.2 g; Cholesterol: 0 mg; Sodium: 83 mg

51.Lean Steak with Healthy Pistachio Pesto

Yield: 4 Servings
Total Time: 15 Minutes
Prep Time: 10 Minutes
Cook Time: 5 Minutes

Ingredients
- 4 (180g) lean beef steaks
- 1 tablespoon extra-virgin olive oil
- 1 cup baby Spinach
- 1 cup rocket
- 1 cup halved cherry tomatoes

Pistachio pesto
- 1/2 cup extra virgin olive oil
- 1/3 cup toasted pistachios
- 1/3 cup toasted almonds
- 1 garlic clove, crushed
- 1/4 cup basil leaves
- 1/2 cup mint leaves
- 1 cup baby rocket

Directions

In a food processor, process together pistachios, garlic, basil, mint, rocket, and toasted almonds until very smooth; add in oil, salt and pepper and continue pulsing until very smooth. Set aside.

Preheat the BBQ grill on medium heat and then brush the meat with oil; season with salt and pepper. Grill for about 3 minutes per side or until cooked to your desire. Transfer to a plate and cover with a plastic wrap.

Slice the steak and divide among the serving plates; top each serving with spinach and tomatoes and season with salt and pepper. Serve with the creamy pistachio pesto.

Nutritional Information per Serving:

Calories: 598; Total Fat: 50 g; Carbs: 4 g; Dietary Fiber: 3 g; Sugars: 2 g; Protein: 33 g; Cholesterol: 218 mg; Sodium: 652 mg

Yield: 4 Servings
Total Time: 25 Minutes
Prep Time: 15 Minutes
Cook Time: 10 Minutes

Ingredients
- 500g lean pork fillet
- 1/4 cup toasted chopped almonds
- 1.2kg pumpkin, diced
- 1 cup baby rocket

Chimichurri
- 2 tablespoons olive oil
- 1 tablespoon raw honey
- 1/4 cup red wine vinegar
- 1/2 cup fresh mint leaves
- 1/3 cup fresh parsley
- 1 cup fresh coriander
- 2 garlic cloves, peeled
- 1 long red chilli, chopped

Directions

Preheat your oven to 400 degrees and line two baking trays with baking paper. Arrange pumpkin on the trays in a single layer; drizzle with olive oil and season with salt and pepper. Bake for about 40 minutes or until golden.

Coat pork with olive oil and season with salt and pepper; heat skillet over medium high heat and cook in the pork for about 5 minutes per side or until cooked to your desire. Wrap in foil and let rest for a few minutes.

Meanwhile, in a food processor, pulse together garlic, chilli, mint, parsley, raw honey, and vinegar until finely chopped; stir in olive oil and season with salt and pepper.

Slice the pork and divide on serving plates; top with pumpkin, almonds and rocket. Drizzle with chimichurri sauce and serve right away.

Nutritional Information per Serving:
Calories: 401; Total Fat: 20 g; Carbs: 15 g; Dietary Fiber: 8 g; Sugars: 9 g; Protein: 35 g; Cholesterol: 112 mg; Sodium: 215 mg

Yield: 4 Servings
Total Time: 30 Minutes
Prep Time: 20 Minutes
Cook Time: 10 Minutes

Ingredients

- 4 (120g each) skinless salmon fillets
- 1 teaspoon dried oregano
- 1 teaspoon onion powder
- 1 teaspoon ground paprika
- 1 teaspoon ground coriander
- 1 teaspoon ground cumin
- 1 tablespoon olive oil
- Thinly shaved fennel
- Baby rocket leaves

Avocado-Mango Salsa

- 1/2 red onion, chopped
- 1 cucumber, chopped
- 1 avocado, diced
- 1 mango, diced
- 1 long red chilli, chopped
- 2 tablespoons lime juice
- 1/2 cup chopped coriander

Directions

In a bowl, mix together onion powder, paprika, coriander, cumin, and oil until well combined; add in salmon and turn until well coated; sprinkle with salt and pepper.
Preheat the BBQ grill on medium high and grill the fish for about 3 minutes per side or until cooked to your liking.
Wrap in foil and let set for at least 5 minutes.
In the meantime, in a bowl, mix together avocado, mango, red onion, cucumber, chilli, coriander, and fresh lime juice until well combined.

Divide fennel and rocket on serving plates and top each with the grilled salmon and mango-avocado salsa. Serve right away.

Nutritional Information per Serving:

Calories: 445; Total Fat: 30 g; Carbs: 17 g; Dietary Fiber: 5 g; Sugars: 12 g; Protein: 29 g; Cholesterol: 107 mg; Sodium: 107 mg

54.Lemon & Garlic Barbecued Ocean Trout

Yield: 8 Servings
Total Time: 40 Minutes
Prep Time: 25 Minutes
Cook Time: 15 Minutes

Ingredients
- 1.5kg piece trout fillet
- 2 tablespoons lemon juice
- 4 garlic cloves, sliced
- 1 long red chilli, sliced
- 2 tablespoons chopped capers
- 1/2 cup fresh parsley
- 1/2 cup olive oil
- Lemon wedges

Directions

Brush the trout with 2 tablespoons of oil and then place it, skin-side up on a barbecue plate. Cook over the preheated barbecue on high for about 5 minutes and then turn it over. Close the hood and cook on medium heat for another 15 minutes or until cooked through. Transfer to a plate.

In a pan, heat the remaining oil and then sauté garlic until lightly browned. Remove from heat and stir in chilli, capers and fresh lemon juice; drizzle over the fish and then sprinkle with parsley. Serve garnished with fresh lemon wedges.

Nutrition information per Serving:

Calories: 420; Total Fat: 30 g; Carbs: 2 g; Dietary Fiber: 1 g; Sugars: 1 g; Protein: 37 g; Cholesterol: 111 mg; Sodium: 160 mg;

Yield: 4 Servings
Total Time: 30 Minutes
Prep Time: 15 Minutes
Cook Time: 15 Minutes

Ingredients

- 8 ounces grilled sardines
- 1 tablespoon canola oil
- 1 large sweet onion, sliced
- 2 tablespoons balsamic vinegar
- ½ cup plain Greek yogurt
- 2 tablespoons white-wine vinegar
- 4 teaspoons minced shallot
- 1 cup halved cherry tomatoes
- 2 hearts romaine, halved lengthwise
- 1 teaspoon salt and pepper

Directions

Heat oil in a pan over medium low heat; add in onions and salt and fry, stirring for about 10 minutes or until the onions are tender and browned. Stir in balsamic vinegar and simmer for about 2 minutes or until the liquid is reduced to a glaze. In a small bowl, make the dressing by whisking together yogurt, shallots, white wine vinegar, pepper and salt. Divide the romaine lettuce among the serving plate and top with the dressing. Top each with grilled sardines and then top with tomatoes and caramelized onions.

Nutrition information per Serving:

Calories: 202; Total Fat: 10g; Carbs: 13 g; Dietary Fiber: 3 g; Sugars: 7 g; Protein: 14 g; Cholesterol: 60 mg; Sodium: 570 mg

56. Herb & Walnut Crusted Salmon

Yield: 4 Servings
Total Time: 25 Minutes
Prep Time: 10 Minutes
Cook Time: 15 Minutes

Ingredients
- 1 (1 pound) skinless fresh salmon fillet
- 2 teaspoons Dijon mustard
- ¼ teaspoon crushed red pepper
- ½ teaspoon raw honey
- 1 teaspoon chopped rosemary
- 1 teaspoon lemon juice
- ¼ teaspoon lemon zest
- 1 clove garlic, minced
- ½ teaspoon kosher salt
- 1 teaspoon extra-virgin olive oil
- 3 tablespoons chopped walnuts
- 3 tablespoons coconut flour
- Chopped fresh parsley

Directions

Preheat your oven to 425 degrees. Prepare a baking sheet by lining it with parchment paper.

In a bowl, combine together crushed red pepper, honey, rosemary, mustard, garlic, fresh lemon juice, lemon zest, and salt until well blended. In another bowl, mix coconut flour, oil and walnuts.

Put the fish on the baking sheet and spread with the herb mixture and then sprinkle with walnut mixture, pressing to adhere. Drizzle with more olive oil and bake in the preheated oven for about 15 minutes or until the fish is cooked through and the outside is golden browned. Serve sprinkled with fresh parsley.

Nutrition information per Serving:

Calories: 222; Total Fat: 12 g; Carbs: 4 g; Dietary Fiber: 0 g; Sugars: 1 g; Protein: 24 g; Cholesterol: 62 mg; Sodium: 256 mg;

57. Delicious Low Carb Chicken Curry

Yield: 1 Serving
Total Time: 30 Minutes
Prep Time: 10 Minutes
Cook Time: 20 Minutes

Ingredients

- 100 grams chicken, diced
- ¼ cup chicken broth
- Pinch of turmeric
- Dash of onion powder
- 1 tablespoon minced red onion
- Pinch of garlic powder
- ¼ teaspoon curry powder
- Pinch of sea salt
- Pinch of pepper
- Stevia, optional
- Pinch of cayenne

Directions

In a small saucepan, stir spices in chicken broth until dissolved; stir in chicken, garlic, onion, and stevia and cook until chicken is cooked through and liquid is reduced by half. Serve hot.

Nutritional Information per Serving:

Calories: 170; Total Fat: 3.5 g; Carbs: 2.3 g; Dietary Fiber: 0.6 g; Sugars: 0.8 g; Protein: 30.5 g; Cholesterol: 77 mg; Sodium: 255 mg

58. Tilapia with Mushroom Sauce

Yields: 4 Servings
Total Time: 35 Minutes
Prep Time: 15 Minutes
Cook Time: 20 Minutes

Ingredients

- 6 ounces tilapia fillets
- 2 teaspoon arrow root
- 1 cup mushrooms, sliced
- 1 clove garlic, finely chopped
- 1 small onion, thinly sliced
- 2 tablespoons extra-virgin olive oil
- ½ cup fresh parsley, roughly chopped
- 1 teaspoon thyme leaves, finely chopped
- ½ cup water
- A pinch of freshly ground black pepper
- A pinch of sea salt

Directions

Preheat your oven to 350°F.

Add extra virgin olive oil to a frying pan set over medium heat; sauté onion, garlic and mushrooms for about 4 minutes or until mushrooms are slightly tender.

Stir in arrowroot, sea salt, thyme and pepper and cook for about 1 minute.

Stir in water until thickened; stir in parsley and cook for 1 minute more.

Place the fillets on a baking tray lined with parchment paper; cover the fish with mushroom sauce and bake for about 20 minutes or until the fish is cooked through.

Nutritional Information per Serving:

Calories: 177; Total Fat: 7.2 g; Carbs: 3.3 g; Dietary Fiber: 1.4 g; Sugars: 1.1 g; Protein: 14.9 g; Cholesterol: 1 mg; Sodium: 66 mg

59.Healthy Roast Salmon with Green Salsa

Yield: 6 Servings
Total Time: 30 Minutes
Prep Time: 15 Minutes
Cook Time: 15 Minutes

Ingredients

- 6 x 200g salmon fillets, skin on
- 3 cups halved cherry tomatoes
- 12 fresh bay leaves
- 2 lemons, sliced
- 6 fresh rosemary sprigs
- 2 tablespoons extra virgin olive oil
- Steamed green beans, to serve

Green Salsa

- 1 tablespoon capers, drained, washed
- 2 tablespoons pitted green olives
- 2 cups mixed fresh herbs (basil, parsley, mint, and chives)
- 1 garlic clove, finely chopped
- 4 tablespoons extra virgin olive oil
- 2 teaspoons white wine vinegar
- 1 teaspoon Dijon mustard

Directions

Preheat your oven to 400 degrees. Sprinkle salmon with salt and pepper and place it on a chopping board, skin side down. Top each fillet with 2 lemon slices, a rosemary sprig and 2 bay leaves; secure with a kitchen string.

In a roasting pan, add tomatoes and drizzle with oil; add in salmon and bake for about 15 minutes or until cooked through. Remove from oven and let rest for at least 5 minutes.
In the meantime, place all salsa ingredients in a food processor and process until chopped. Divide the salmon and tomatoes among serving plates and top each with beans and green salsa. Enjoy!

Nutrition information per Serving:

Calories: 554; Total Fat: 42 g; Carbs: 8.3 g; Dietary Fiber: 2.9 g; Sugars: 3.8 g; Protein: 40.4 g; Cholesterol: 370 mg; Sodium: 84 mg;

60. Ginger Chicken with Veggies

Yields: 4 Servings
Total Time: 15 Minutes
Prep Time: 10 Minutes
Cook Time: 5 Minutes

Ingredients

- 2 cup skinless, boneless, and cooked chicken breast meat, diced
- ¼ cup extra virgin olive and canola oil mixture
- 1 teaspoon powdered ginger
- ½ red onion, sliced
- 2 cloves garlic, minced
- ½ bell pepper, sliced
- 1 cup thinly sliced carrots
- ½ cup finely chopped celery
- 1 cup chicken broth (not salted)

Directions

Add the oil mixture to a skillet set over medium heat; sauté onion and garlic until translucent. Stir in the remaining ingredients and simmer for a few minutes or until the veggies are tender.

Nutritional Info per Serving:

Calories: 425; Fat: 21.1g; Carbs: 6.5 g; Dietary Fiber: 3.2 g; Sugars: 1.1 g; Protein: 52g; Cholesterol: 107 mg; Sodium: 110 mg

61. Tangy Whole Roasted Sea Bass with Oregano

Yield: 4 Servings
Total Time: 35 Minutes
Prep Time: 15 Minutes
Cook Time: 20 Minutes

Ingredients

- 2 medium-sized whole sea bass
- 1 tbsp. extra virgin olive oil
- 2 garlic cloves, thinly sliced
- ½ tsp. dried oregano
- 2 tsp. freshly squeezed lemon juice
- Kosher salt and freshly ground pepper, to taste
- 2 lemons, thinly sliced

Directions

Start by preheating your broiler or grill to medium-high heat. Lightly grease the rack with olive oil cooking spray.

Combine the lemon juice, olive oil, salt, pepper and oregano in a bowl and let stand. Use a sharp knife to make 3 horizontal slits on each side of the fish and rub with some kosher salt. Use a brush to rub in the lemon-herb mixture in the slits.

Cook the fish in the reheated broiler/ grill for about 15-20 minutes, turning twice in between cook time and baste with the lemon-oregano mixture. Grill until the flesh turns opaque or until desired doneness is achieved.

Let the sea bass rest for 50-10 minutes before serving. Serve with steamed veggies or a salad.

Enjoy!

Nutritional Information per Serving:

Calories: 236; Total Fat: 16g; Carbs: 2g; Dietary Fiber 1g; Protein: 37g; Cholesterol: 0mg; Sodium: 563mg

62.Ground Beef Lettuce Tacos

Yield: 1 Serving
Total Time: 35 Minutes
Prep Time: 10 Minutes
Cook Time: 25 Minutes

Ingredients

- 100 grams lean ground beef
- 1 clove garlic, minced
- ½ red onion, minced
- Lettuce leaves
- Cayenne pepper
- Fresh chopped cilantro
- Pinch of dried oregano
- Dash of onion powder
- Dash of garlic powder
- Pinch of salt & pepper

Directions:

Fry beef in a splash of lemon juice until browned; add garlic, onion and spices, and water and simmer for about 5-10 minutes. Season with salt and serve taco style in romaine lettuce or butter lettuce or with a side of salsa or tomatoes.

Nutritional Information per Serving:

Calories: 194; Total Fat: 6.3 g; Carbs: 1.9 g; Dietary Fiber: 0.5 g; Sugars: 0.7 g; Protein: 30.6 g; Cholesterol: 89 mg; Sodium: 67 mg

63.Pepper Crusted Steak

Yield: 1 Serving
Total Time: 15 Minutes
Prep Time: 10 Minutes
Cook Time: 5 Minutes

Ingredients

- 100 grams lean steak
- Dash of Worcestershire sauce
- Pinch of salt & pepper

Directions:

Pound meat until tender and flat; rub with salt and pepper and cook on high heat for about 3-5 minutes. Serve topped with Worcestershire sauce and garnished with caramelized onions.

Nutritional Information per Serving:

Calories: 189; Total Fat: 6.2 g; Carbs: 0.2 g; Dietary Fiber: 0 g; Sugars: 0.1 g; Protein: 30.4 g; Cholesterol: 89 mg; Sodium: 228 mg

64.Ginger Chicken with Veggies

Yields: 4 Servings
Total Time: 15 Minutes
Prep Time: 10 Minutes
Cook Time: 5 Minutes

Ingredients

- 2 cup skinless, boneless, and cooked chicken breast meat, diced
- ¼ cup extra virgin olive and canola oil mixture
- 1 teaspoon powdered ginger
- ½ red onion, sliced
- 2 cloves garlic, minced
- ½ bell pepper, sliced
- 1 cup thinly sliced carrots
- ½ cup finely chopped celery
- 1 cup chicken broth (not salted)

Directions

Add the oil mixture to a skillet set over medium heat; sauté onion and garlic until translucent. Stir in the remaining ingredients and simmer for a few minutes or until the veggies are tender.

Nutritional Info per Serving:

Calories: 425; Fat: 21.1g; Carbs: 6.5 g; Dietary Fiber: 3.2 g; Sugars: 1.1 g; Protein: 52g; Cholesterol: 107 mg; Sodium: 110 mg

65.Curried Goat Stew

Yield: 4 Servings
Total Time: 7-8 Hours
Prep Time: 15 Minutes
Cook Time: 7-8 Hours

Ingredients
- 8 goat chops
- 2 tbsp. olive oil or coconut oil
- 6 carrots, cut in 2-inch pieces
- 1 sweet onion, cut in thin wedges
- 1 cup unsweetened coconut milk
- 1/4 cup mild (or hot) curry paste
- Toasted almonds, coriander and fresh green or red chili

Directions

Cook the chops in a pan in hot oil for 8 minutes, or until browned. Remove from heat; drain and discard fat.

In a slow cooker combine carrots and onion. Whisk together half the coconut milk and the Curry paste then pour over carrots and onion. Place the goat meat on top of vegetables and pour over oil from pan.

Cover and cook on low for 7 to 8 hours.

Remove chops from the pot. Remove excess fat from sauce and stir in remaining coconut milk.

Once cooled, transfer to freezer bags or jars and freeze until you are ready to eat.

When serving, top with chopped toasted almonds and a dollop of plain Greek yogurt.

Nutritional Information per Serving:

Calories: 602; Total Fat: 38.1 g; Carbs: 21.1 g; Dietary Fiber: 5.6 g; Sugars: 8.8 g; Protein: 59.8 g; Cholesterol: 309 mg; Sodium: 654 mg

66.   Creamy Coconut Sardines Escabeche

Yield: 6 Servings
Total Time: 48 Minutes
Prep Time: 20 Minutes
Cook Time: 38 Minutes

Ingredients
- 1kg fresh sardines
- 150ml extra virgin olive oil
- 1 red onion, thinly sliced
- 1 carrot, thinly sliced
- 2 garlic cloves, thinly sliced
- 4 tablespoons sherry vinegar
- 2 cups coconut milk
- ½ cup coconut cream
- 2 tablespoons chopped flat-leaf parsley
- 2 fresh bay leaves
- 1 teaspoon black peppercorns
- 3-4 thyme sprigs
- 1 teaspoon cumin seeds
- 3 tablespoons almond flour

Directions

Wash the sardines with warm water and dry with paper towel; mix flour with salt and pepper and then dust the sardines with the flour.

Heat half of the oil in a pan set over medium heat and cook the sardines in batches for about 5 minutes per side or until cooked through and lightly browned; transfer to a dish and clean the pan, add in the remaining oil and sauté the onions for about 4 minutes or until lightly browned; stir in garlic and carrots and cook for another minute. Stir in the coconut milk along with remaining ingredients and simmer for about 5 minutes or until liquid is by half; add in sardines and stir to coat well. Cook for about 2 minutes and then remove from heat. Serve with brown rice.

Nutrition information per Serving:

Calories: 568; Total Fat: 41 g; Carbs: 7 g; Dietary Fiber: 2 g; Sugars: 2 g; Protein: 41 g; Cholesterol: 108 mg; Sodium: 84 mg;

67.Beef Stir Fry with Red Onions & Cabbage

Yield: 4 Servings
Total Time: 20 Minutes
Prep Time: 10 Minutes
Cook Time: 10 Minutes

Ingredients:

- 550g grass-fed flank steak, thinly sliced strips
- 1 tablespoon apple cider wine
- 2 teaspoons balsamic vinegar
- Pinch of sea salt
- pinch of pepper
- 4 tablespoons extra-virgin olive oil
- 1 large yellow onion, thinly chopped
- 1/2 red bell pepper, thinly sliced
- 1/2 green bell pepper, thinly sliced
- 1 tablespoon toasted sesame seeds
- 1 teaspoon crushed red pepper flakes
- 4 cups cabbage
- 1 ½ avocados, diced

Directions:

Place meat in a bowl; stir in rice wine and vinegar, sea salt and pepper. Toss to coat well. Heat a tablespoon of olive oil in a pan set over medium high heat; add meat and cook for about 2 minutes or until meat is browned; stir for another 2 minutes and then remove from heat. Heat the remaining oil to the pan and sauté onions for about 2 minutes or until caramelized; stir in pepper and cook for 2 minutes more. Stir in cabbage and cook for 2 minutes; return meat to pan and stir in sesame seeds and red pepper flakes. Serve hot topped with diced avocado!

Nutritional Info per Serving:

Calories: 459; Fat: 30 g; Carbs: 16.6 g; Dietary Fiber: 6.1 g; Sugars: 7.8 g; Protein: 35.3 g; Cholesterol: 112 mg; Sodium: 516 mg

68.Spiced Roast Side of Salmon

Yield: 6 Servings
Total Time: 30 Minutes
Prep Time: 10 Minutes
Cook Time: 20 Minutes

Ingredients
- 1 tablespoon olive oil
- 1½ kg side of salmon
- 1 teaspoon honey
- 1 tablespoon wholegrain mustard
- ½ teaspoon black peppercorns
- 1 teaspoon paprika
- ½ teaspoon ground ginger
- 1 lemon, cut into wedges

Directions

Preheat your oven to 350 degrees and prepare a roasting tin by lining it with foil. Brush the fish with oil and place in the tin, skin side down.

In a small bowl, mix together a teaspoon of olive oil, honey, mustard, pepper and paprika and then smear the mixture onto the salmon.

Roast the fish in the oven for 20 minutes or until cooked through. Serve with lemon wedges. Enjoy!

Nutritional Information per Serving:

Calories: 482; Total Fat: 30 g; Carbs: 2 g; Dietary Fiber: 0 g; Sugars: 1 g; Protein: 51 g; Cholesterol: 0 mg; Sodium: 400 mg

69.Coconut-Crumbed Chicken Bake

Yield: 4 Servings
Total Time: 1 Hour 15 Minutes
Prep Time: 15 Minutes
Cook Time: 1 Hour

Ingredients

- 4 skinless chicken breasts
- 1 large aborigine, diced
- 1 butternut squash, diced
- 4 tbsp. gluten-free breadcrumb
- 3 tbsp. desiccated coconut
- 1 tbsp. rapeseed oil
- 2 tbsp. red curry paste
- 300g cherry tomato
- 1 egg, beaten
- lime wedges
- handful coriander, chopped

Directions

Preheat oven to 400°F.
Toss together oil, aubergine, and squash in a large bowl; spread out in a roasting pan and roast for about 30 minutes, turning once. Mix bread crumbs, coconut and some seasoning on a plate; dip chicken in egg and then press into the crumb mixture.

Stir curry paste and tomatoes in the roasted veggies and nestle chicken in the center of the veggies; bake in the oven for about 30 minutes or until chicken is cooked through. Serve garnished with lime wedges and coriander.

Nutritional Info per Serving:

Calories: 477; Total Fat: 22.7 g; Carbs: 19.8 g; Dietary Fiber: 4.3 g; Sugars: 5.2 g; Protein: 45.9 g; Cholesterol: 171 mg; Sodium: 586 mg

Yield: 4 Servings
Total Time: 27 Minutes
Prep Time: 15 Minutes
Cook Time: 12 Minutes

Ingredients

- 400g raw king prawns
- 1 tablespoon vegetable oil
- 40g ginger, grated
- 2-4 green chillies, halved
- 4 curry leaves
- 1 onion, sliced
- 4 teaspoons lemon juice
- 3-4 teaspoons red chilli powder
- 2 teaspoons turmeric
- 1 teaspoon black pepper
- 40g grated coconut
- ½ small bunch coriander

Directions

Rinse the prawns and pat dry with a kitchen towel; add them to a large bowl and then toss in chili powder, turmeric, grated ginger, and lemon juice; set aside.

Heat oil in a saucepan and sauté onion, ginger, chilli, and curry leaves for about 10 minutes or until translucent. Stir in black pepper and then add in prawns along with the marinade. Cook for about 2 minutes or until cooked through. Season and drizzle with extra lemon juice. Serve the prawns sprinkled with coriander and grated coconut. Enjoy!

Nutritional Information per Serving:

Calories: 171; Total Fat: 8 g; Carbs: 4 g; Dietary Fiber: 3 g; Sugars: 1 g; Protein: 19 g; Cholesterol: 0 mg; Sodium: 802 mg

71.Delicious Chicken Tikka Skewers

Yield: 4 Servings
Total Time: 40 Minutes
Prep Time: 20 Minutes
Cook Time: 20 Minutes

Ingredients
- 4 boneless, skinless chicken breasts, diced
- 2 tablespoons hot curry paste
- 1 red onion, sliced
- ½ cucumber, sliced
- For the cucumber salad
- 250g pack cherry tomatoes
- 50g pack lamb's lettuce
- juice 1 lemon
- 150g natural yogurt
- handful chopped coriander leaves

Directions

Soak skewers in a bowl of water.

In a bowl, mix together curry paste and yogurt; add in chicken and then marinate for 1 hour.

Meanwhile, toss together red onion, cucumber, coriander, and fresh lemon juice in a bowl. Refrigerate until ready to serve.

Thread chicken and cherry tomatoes on the skewers and grill for about 20 minutes or until cooked through and golden browned on the outside.

Add the lettuce into the salad and stir in mix well; divide among serving bowls and top each with two chicken skewers. Enjoy!

Nutritional Information per Serving:

Calories: 234; Total Fat: 4 g; Carbs: 9.7 g; Dietary Fiber: 2.7 g; Sugars: 8.3g; Protein: 40 g; Cholesterol: 394 mg; Sodium: 773 mg

72.Stir-Fried Chicken with Water Chestnuts

Yield: 4 Servings
Total Time: 25 Minutes
Prep Time: 10 Minutes
Cook Time: 15 Minutes

Ingredients

- 2 tablespoons sesame oil
- ¼ cup wheat-free tamari
- 4 small chicken breasts, sliced
- 1 small cabbage, chopped
- 3 garlic cloves, chopped
- ¼ teaspoons peppercorns
- ¼ teaspoon ground fennel seeds
- 1/4 teaspoon cinnamon
- 1/4 teaspoon ground cloves
- ¼ teaspoon star anise
- 1 cup dried plums
- 1 cup water chestnuts
- Toasted sesame seeds

Directions

Heat sesame oil in a large skillet set over medium heat; stir in all the ingredients, except sesame seeds, and cook until cabbage and chicken are tender.
Serve warm sprinkled with toasted sesame seeds.

Nutritional Information per Serving:

Calories: 306; Total Fat: 13.5 g; Carbs: 23.4 g; Dietary Fiber: 0.7 g; Sugars: 2 g; Protein: 22.5 g; Cholesterol: 62 mg; Sodium: 29 mg

73.Pan-Fried Chili Beef with Toasted Cashews

Yields: 4 Servings
Total Time: 35 Minutes
Prep Time: 10 Minutes
Cook Time: 25 Minutes

Ingredients

- ½ tablespoon extra-virgin olive oil or canola oil
- 1 pound sliced lean beef
- 2 teaspoons red curry paste
- 1 teaspoon raw honey
- 2 tablespoons fresh lime juice
- 2 teaspoon fish sauce
- 1 cup green capsicum, diced
- ½ cup water
- 24 toasted cashews
- 1 teaspoon arrowroot

Directions

Add oil to a pan set over medium heat; add beef and fry until its no longer pink inside. Stir in red curry paste and cook for a few more minutes.
Stir in honey, lime juice, fish sauce, capsicum and water; simmer for about 10 minutes.
Mix cooked arrowroot with water to make a paste; stir the paste into the sauce to thicken it.
Remove the pan from heat and add the fried cashews. Serve.

Nutritional Information per Serving:

Calories: 361; Total Fat: 17.7 g; Carbs: 12.9 g; Dietary Fiber: 1.2 g; Sugars: 3.8 g; Protein: 38 g; Cholesterol: 101 mg; Sodium: 444 mg

74.Healthy Keto Coconut-Lime Skirt Steak

Yield: 4 Servings
Total Time: 40 Minutes
Prep Time: 10 Minutes
Cook Time: 30 Minutes

Ingredients:
- 2 pounds skirt steak, cut into sections
- 2 tbsp. fresh lime juice
- 1/2 cup melted coconut oil
- 1 tsp red pepper flakes
- 1 tsp grated fresh ginger
- 1 tbsp. minced garlic
- zest of one lime
- 3/4 tsp sea salt

Directions

In a bowl, mix together lime juice, coconut oil, red pepper flakes, ginger, garlic, lime zest and salt until well combined.
Toss in steak and marinate for at least 20 minutes; transfer the meat to a skillet set over medium heat and spoon over the marinade.
Sear the meat for about 5 minutes per side or until cooked through and golden brown.
Serve and enjoy!

Nutritional Information per Serving:

Calories: 661; Total Fat: 54g; Carbs: 5g; Dietary Fiber: 0g; Sugars: 1g; Protein: 35g; Cholesterol: Sodium:

75.Healthy Low-Carb Grilled Turkey

Yield: 12 Servings
Total Time: 50 Minutes
Prep Time: 15 Minutes
Cook Time: 35 Minutes

Ingredients

- 5 pounds turkey breast cutlets
- 3 tbsp. extra virgin olive oil
- 1-1/2 teaspoons garlic powder
- 1-1/2 teaspoons sweet paprika
- 2 tsp. crushed fennel seeds
- 1 teaspoon sea salt
- 1-1/2 teaspoons freshly ground black pepper

Directions

Mix together garlic powder, paprika, fennel seeds, salt and pepper in a small bowl; rub the mixture over the turkey meat.

Add 3 tablespoons of olive oil to a skillet and heat over medium heat; add turkey meat and cook until browned on both sides.

Transfer the grilled turkey to a serving plate and let rest for about 5 minutes. Serve.

Nutritional Information per Serving

Calories: 258; Total Fat: 9.1 g; Carbs: 0.5 g; Dietary fiber: 0.2 g; Sugars: 0 g; Protein: 24 g; Cholesterol: 100 mg; Sodium: 334 mg

76.Lemon-pepper BBQ fish with greens and salsa

Yield: 4 Servings
Total Time: 20 Minutes
Prep Time: 10 Minutes
Cook Time: 10 Minutes

Ingredients
- 4 white fish fillets
- 2 bunches asparagus, ends removed
- 2 bunches baby broccoli, ends removed
- 1 red onion, finely chopped
- 2 large tomatoes, finely chopped
- 2 tablespoons shredded mint leaves
- 2 tablespoons chopped capers
- 1 green chilli, seeded, finely chopped
- 1 teaspoon lemon zest
- 1 teaspoon black pepper
- 1 tablespoon olive oil
- 1/2 teaspoons salt

Directions

In a bowl, mix together oil, mint, capers, chilli, red onion, and tomatoes; season with salt and pepper and set aside.

In a small bowl, mix together lemon zest, pepper and salt; sprinkle over the fish until well coated.

Heat the BBQ grill on medium high heat and spray the asparagus and broccoli with olive oil; season with salt and pepper; grill for about 2 minutes per side or until crisp and charred. Transfer to a plate and keep warm.

Drizzle fish with olive oil and grill for about 3 minutes per side or until cooked through and golden browned on both sides. Divide the asparagus and broccoli on serving plates and top each with the tomato mixture and grilled fish.

Nutritional Information per Serving:

Calories: 223; Total Fat: 7 g; Carbs: 5 g; Dietary Fiber: 7 g; Sugars: 4 g; Protein: 31 g; Cholesterol: 112 mg; Sodium: 534 mg

Gestational Diabetes Snacks/Desserts

77.Healthy Nutty Guacamole

Yield: 8 Servings
Total Time: 20 Minutes
Prep Time: 10 Minutes
Cook Time: 10 Minutes

Ingredients
- ½ cup chopped pistachios
- ½ cup chopped walnuts
- ½ cup chopped almonds
- 1 tablespoon olive oil
- 4 ripe avocados
- 1 cup chopped shallots
- 1 cup chopped tomatoes
- 1/2 cup fresh lemon juice
- 1 teaspoon raw honey
- ½ teaspoon sea salt

Directions

Heat olive oil in a skillet and toasted in walnuts, almonds and pistachios until well toasted. In a large bowl, mash together diced avocado, shallots, tomatoes, lime juice, raw honey, and sea salt until well blended. Stir in the toasted nuts to combine well and then serve right away.

Nutrition Information per Serving:

Calories: 347; Total Fat: 30.9 g; Carbs: 17 g; Dietary Fiber: 8.7 g; Sugar: 2.7 g; Protein: 6.6 g; Cholesterol: 0 mg; Sodium: 150 mg

78.Sesame Crackers

Yields: 96 Crackers
Total Time: 32 Minutes
Prep Time: 20 Minutes
Cook Time: 12 Minutes

Ingredients

- 1 cup sesame seeds
- 2 tbsp. grapeseed oil
- 2 large free range eggs, beaten
- 1 ½ tsp. sea salt
- 3 cups almond flour, blanched

Directions

Stir together sesame seeds, almond flour, oil, eggs and salt in a large bowl until well combined.
Divide the dough into two portions.
Place each into two baking sheets lined with parchment papers and cover with parchment paper.
Spread the dough between the papers to cover the entire baking sheet and remove the top paper.

With a pizza cutter or knife, cut the dough into 2-inch squares and bake at 350°F until golden brown, for about 12 minutes.
Cool before serving.

Nutritional Information per Serving:

Calories: 178; Total Fat: 15.6 g; Carbs: 6 g; Dietary Fiber: 3.3 g; Protein: 6.1 g; Cholesterol: 20 mg; Sodium: 184 mg

79.Roasted Asparagus

Yield: 4 Servings
Total Time: 15 Minutes
Prep Time: 5 Minutes
Cook Time: 10 Minutes

Ingredients

- 1 tbsp. extra virgin olive oil
- 1 pound fresh asparagus
- 1 medium lemon, zested
- 1/2 tsp. freshly grated nutmeg
- 1/2 tsp. kosher salt
- ½ tsp. black pepper

Directions

Preheat your oven to 500°F. Arrange asparagus on an aluminum foil and drizzle with extra virgin olive oil; toss until well coated. Spread the asparagus in a single layer and fold the edges of foil to make a tray. Roast the asparagus in the oven for about 5 minutes; toss and continue roasting for 5 minutes more or until browned. Sprinkle the roasted asparagus with nutmeg, salt, zest and pepper to serve.

Nutritional Information per Serving:

Calories: 55; Total Fat: 3.8 g; Carbs: 4.7 g; Dietary Fiber: 2.5 g; Protein: 2.5 g; Cholesterol: 0 mg; Sodium: 293 mg

Yield: 8 Servings
Total Time: 10 Minutes
Prep Time: 10 Minutes
Cook Time: N/A

Ingredients

- 2 cup peanuts roasted
- 1 teaspoon red chili powder
- 2 tablespoons cilantro
- 1 teaspoon lemon juice
- 1 teaspoon chai masala
- 1/2 cup chopped tomato
- 1/2 cup chopped onion
- 1 teaspoon salt

Directions

Mix all ingredients in a large bowl until well combined. Serve.

Nutritional Information per Serving:

Calories: 420; Total Fat: 35.2 g; Carbs: 16.5 g; Dietary Fiber: 6.1 g; Sugars: 3.6 g; Protein: 17 g; Cholesterol: 0 mg; Sodium: 871 mg

81.Turmeric Coconut Latte

Yield: 1 Serving
Total Time: 15 Minutes
Prep Time: 10 Minutes
Cook Time: 5 Minutes

Ingredients
- 1 cup unsweetened coconut milk
- 1 teaspoon grated fresh ginger
- 1 teaspoon stevia
- 1 tablespoon grated fresh turmeric
- A pinch of cinnamon
- A pinch of ground pepper

Directions

In a blender, blend together milk, ginger, stevia, turmeric, and pepper until very smooth; pour into a pan and cook until just heated through. Transfer to a mag and serve sprinkled with cinnamon. Enjoy!

Nutrition information per Serving:

Calories: 70; Total Fat: 3 g; Carbs: 11 g; Dietary Fiber: 1 g; Sugars: 8 g; Protein: 1 g; Cholesterol: 0 mg; Sodium: 172 mg

82.Delicious Ginger Tahini Dip

Yield: 8 Servings
Total Time: 5 Minutes
Prep Time: 5 Minutes
Cook Time: N/A

Ingredients
- ½ cup tahini
- 1 teaspoon grated garlic
- 2 teaspoons ground turmeric
- 1 tablespoon grated fresh ginger
- ¼ cup apple cider vinegar
- ¼ cup water
- ½ teaspoon salt

Directions

In a bowl, whisk together tahini, turmeric, ginger, water, vinegar, garlic, and salt until well blended. Serve with assorted veggies.

Nutrition information per Serving:

Calories: 92; Total Fat: 8 g; Carbs: 4 g; Dietary Fiber: 1 g; Sugars: 0 g; Protein: 3 g; Cholesterol: 0 mg; Sodium: 151 mg;

Yield: 1 Serving
Total Time: 10 Minutes
Prep Time: 10 Minutes
Cook Time: N/A

Ingredient

- 1 tablespoon extra-virgin olive oil
- 1/4 cup toasted sesame tahini
- 1/4 cup apple cider vinegar
- 1/2 cup chickpeas
- 1 clove garlic, minced
- 1/2 teaspoon ground cumin
- ½ teaspoon red chili powder
- 1 teaspoon sea salt
- 3 tablespoons water

Directions

In a food processor, combine all ingredients and pulse until very smooth. Serve with carrots or cucumber slices.

Nutritional Information per Serving:

Calories: 106; Total Fat: 6.1 g; Carbs: 10.3 g; Dietary Fiber: 6.9 g; Sugars: 1.7g; Protein: 4.3 g; Cholesterol: 0 mg; Sodium: 221 mg

84.Spiced & Sweet Lassi

Yield: 6 Servings
Total Time: 5 Minutes
Prep Time: 5 Minutes
Cook Time: N/A

Ingredients

- 3 cups yogurt
- 3 cups water
- 1 tablespoon toasted cumin seeds
- 1 tablespoon chopped coriander

Directions

In a blender, whisk together yogurt and water until frothy. Stir in toasted cumin seeds and chopped coriander. Enjoy!

Nutritional Information per Serving:

Calories: 91; Total Fat: 1.7 g; Carbs: 9.1 g; Dietary Fiber: 0.1 g; Sugars: 8.6 g; Protein: 7.2 g; Cholesterol: 7 mg; Sodium: 91 mg

85.Spiced Spinach Bites

Yield: 4 Servings
Total Time: 1 Hour 15 Minutes
Prep Time: 10 Minutes
Cook Time: 20 Minutes

Ingredients

- 12 baby spinach leaves
- 2 chopped limes
- ½ chopped chilli
- 1 sliced shallot
- 1 teaspoon chopped ginger
- 2 tablespoons peanuts
- A pinch of sea salt
- 1 tablespoon coriander

Directions

In a bowl, combine peanuts, chilli, shallot, ginger, limes, and coriander; season with a sprinkle of sea salt.

Lay spinach leaves on a plate and add a spoonful of the mixture on each; roll them up to make round wraps.

Nutritional Info per Serving:

Calories: 46; Total Fat: 2.5 g; Carbs: 6.1 g; Dietary Fiber: 2.1 g; Sugars: 0.9 g; Protein: 2.4 g; Cholesterol: 0 mg; Sodium: 40 mg

Yields: 12 Servings
Total Time: 35 Minutes
Prep Time: 5 Minutes
Cook Time: 20 Minutes

Ingredients

- 1 teaspoon extra-virgin olive oil
- 1 teaspoon fresh lemon juice
- 1 teaspoon grated lemon peel
- 1 teaspoon crushed red pepper flakes
- 2 sprigs fresh rosemary
- 3 cups mixed olives
- Lemon twists, optional

Directions

Preheat your oven to 400°F. Place pepper flakes, lemon juice, rosemary, olives and grated lemon peel onto a large sheet of foil; drizzle with oil and fold the foil. Pinch the edges of the sheet to tightly seal.

Bake in the preheated oven for about 30 minutes. Remove from the sheet and place the mixture to serving dish. Serve warm garnished with lemon twists.

Nutritional Information per Serving:

Calories: 43; Total Fat: 4 g; Carbs: 2.2 g; Dietary Fiber: 1.1 g; Protein: 0.3 g; Cholesterol: 0 mg; Sodium: 293 mg; Sugars: trace

Yield: 4 Servings
Total Time: 15 Minutes
Prep Time: 5 Minutes
Cook Time: 10 Minutes

Ingredients

- 1 tbsp. extra virgin olive oil
- 1 pound fresh asparagus
- 1 medium lemon, zested
- 1/2 tsp. freshly grated nutmeg
- 1/2 tsp. kosher salt
- ½ tsp. black pepper

Directions

Preheat your oven to 500°F. Arrange asparagus on an aluminum foil and drizzle with extra virgin olive oil; toss until well coated. Spread the asparagus in a single layer and fold the edges of foil to make a tray. Roast the asparagus in the oven for about 5 minutes; toss and continue roasting for 5 minutes more or until browned. Sprinkle the roasted asparagus with nutmeg, salt, zest and pepper to serve.

Nutritional Information per Serving:

Calories: 55; Total Fat: 3.8 g; Carbs: 4.7 g; Dietary Fiber: 2.5 g; Protein: 2.5 g; Cholesterol: 0 mg; Sodium: 293 mg

88.Roasted Spiced Pumpkin Seeds

Yield: 4 Servings
Total Time: 25 Minutes
Prep Time: 5 Minutes
Cook Time: 20 Minutes

Ingredients

- 1 cup shelled pumpkin seeds
- 2 tablespoons fresh lime juice
- 1 teaspoon chili powder
- Coarse salt

Directions

Preheat oven to 350°F.
Toss pumpkin seeds with fresh lime juice, chili powder and sea salt until well coated; spread over a baking sheet and bake for about 20 minutes, stirring once. Remove from oven and let cool before serving.

Nutritional Information per Serving:

Calories: 189; Total Fat: 15.9 g; Carbs: 6.7 g; Dietary Fiber: 1.6 g; Sugars: 0.5 g; Protein: 8.6 g; Cholesterol: 0 mg; Sodium: 13 mg

89.Spiced Apple Crisps

Yield: 4 Servings
Total Time: 35 Minutes
Prep Time: 1 Minutes
Cook Time: 25 Minutes

Ingredients
- 4 apples, slices
- 1 teaspoon liquid stevia
- ½ teaspoon sea salt
- 2 teaspoon cinnamon
- 1 cup virgin olive oil
- 1 teaspoon black pepper

Directions

In a large bowl, stir together cinnamon, stevia, black pepper and sea salt until well blended; add the apple slices into the mixture and toss to coat well.

Heat olive oil in a skillet over medium heat; add in the apple slices and deep fry until golden browned. Drain the apple crisps onto paper towel lined plates and serve with a cup of tea.

Nutritional Information per Serving:

Calories: 413 Total Fat: 21.3 g; Net Carbs: 26 g; Dietary Fiber: 6.8 g; Sugars: 22.3 g; Protein: 3.9 g; Cholesterol: 0 mg; Sodium: 321 mg

90.Amaranth Pop Corns

Yield: 2 Servings
Total Time: 15 Minutes
Prep Time: 5 Minutes
Cook Time: 10 Minutes

Ingredients
- 1/2 cup amaranth seeds
- 1 teaspoon olive oil
- 1 teaspoon cinnamon
- ½ teaspoon sea salt

Directions

Heat olive oil in a pot set over high heat; add in the amaranth seeds and cook until they start popping. Cover the pot and let all seeds pops.
Serve sprinkled with cinnamon and sea salt.

Nutritional Information per Serving:

Calories: 205 Total Fat: 5.5 g; Net Carbs: 28.1 g; Dietary Fiber: 5.1 g; Sugars: 0.8 g; Protein: 7.1 g; Cholesterol: 0 mg; Sodium: 478 mg

91.Healthy Taro Chips

Yield: 4 Servings
Total Time: 30 Minutes
Prep Time: 10 Minutes
Cook Time: 20 Minutes

Ingredients

- 1 pound taro peeled
- 1 teaspoon olive oil
- A pinch of salt
- A pinch of pepper

Directions

With a mandolin, slice the taro lengthwise; place the taro slices on a paper-lined baking sheets and brush with olive oil. Sprinkle with sea salt and pepper and bake at 400 degrees for about 20 minutes or until crisp.

Nutritional Information per Serving:

Calories: 137 Total Fat: 1.4 g; Net Carbs: 25.3 g; Dietary Fiber: 4.7 g; Sugars: 0.5 g; Protein: 1.7 g; Cholesterol: 0 mg; Sodium: 51 mg

92.Crispy Lemon- Chili Roasted Kale

Yield: 2 Servings
Total Time: 30 Minutes
Prep Time: 10 Minutes
Cook Time: 20 Minutes

Ingredients

- 2 bunches kale, ribs and stems removed, roughly chopped
- 2 tablespoons lemon juice
- 2 tablespoons extra-virgin olive oil
- 1 teaspoon lemon salt
- 2 teaspoons chili powder
- Parmesan wedge

Directions

Preheat oven to 250°F.

In a large bowl, massage together kale, lemon juice, extra virgin olive oil, lemon salt and chili powder until kale is tender; spread the kale on a baking sheet and bake for about 20 minutes or until crisp tender. Remove from oven and sprinkle with parmesan cheese. Serve warm.

Nutrition info Per Serving:

Calories: 165; Total Fat: 14.6 g; Carbs: 8.7 g; Dietary Fiber: 2 g; Sugars: 0.5 g; Protein: 2.4 g; Cholesterol: 0 mg; Sodium: 58 mg

93.Heart-Healthy Fats Smoothie

Yield: 4 Servings
Total Time: 5 Minutes
Prep Time: 5 Minutes

Ingredients
- 1 avocado
- 2 cup spinach
- 2 cups diced cucumber
- 1 cup coconut water
- 1 cup chopped cashews
- 4 tablespoons almond butter
- 1 tablespoon hemp seeds
- 4 tablespoons flaxseed
- 1 teaspoon stevia

Directions
Combine all ingredients in a blender; blend until very smooth. Enjoy!

Nutrition Information per Serving:
Calories: 420; Total Fat: 32.1 g; Carbs: 18.5 g; Dietary Fiber: 8.1 g; Sugar: 9.1 g; Protein: 10.8 g; Cholesterol: 0 mg; Sodium: 87 mg

94.Gingery Lemonade

Serving Total: 4 servings
Total Time: 12 Minutes
Prep Time: 5 Minutes
Cook Time: 7 Minutes

Ingredients:
- 14 slices fresh ginger root
- 4 quarts water
- 1 teaspoon stevia
- 4 cups fresh lemon juice
- 2 lemons, sliced

Directions

Combine ginger root, water and stevia in a saucepan set over medium heat.
Bring to a gentle boil.

Remove from heat and stir in lemon juice.
Let cool for about 15 minutes and chill for at least 1 hour.
Serve over ice garnished with lemon slices.

Nutritional Information per Serving:

Calories: 98; Total Fat: 2.1 g; Carbs: 8.2 g; Dietary Fiber: 1.1 g; Protein: 1.1 g; Cholesterol: 0 mg; Sodium: 76 mg; sugars: 9.4 g

Yield: 10 Fudge fat bombs
Total Time: 4 Hours 20 Minutes
Prep Time: 20 Minutes
Cooking Time: N/A

Ingredients

- 1/2 cup coconut oil
- 4 oz. food-grade cocoa butter
- 4 tablespoons unsweetened cocoa powder
- 1/3 cup heavy cream
- 1/2 cup pecans, roughly chopped
- 4 tablespoons erythritol/Swerve

Directions

Melt coconut oil and cocoa butter in a double boiler; whisk in cocoa powder until very smooth and then transfer the mixture to a blender. Add in the sweetener and blend until very smooth. Add in cream and continue blending for about 5 minutes.
Arrange molds onto a sheet pan and fill each half with the pecans; top each with the chocolate mixture and freeze for about 4 hours or until firm.

Nutritional Information per Serving

Calories: 494; Total Fat: 53.1 g; Carbs: 5.2 g; Dietary fiber: 2.2 g; Sugars: 0.9 g; Protein: 2.5 g; Cholesterol: 11 mg; Sodium: 4 mg

96.Roasted Chili-Vinegar Peanuts

Yield: 4 Servings
Total Time: 10 Minutes
Prep Time: 10 Minutes
Cook Time: N/A

Ingredients

- 1 tablespoon coconut oil
- 2 cups raw peanuts, unsalted
- 2 teaspoon sea salt
- 2 tablespoon apple cider vinegar
- 1 teaspoon chili powder
- 1 teaspoon fresh lime zest

Directions

Preheat oven to 350°F.

In a large bowl, toss together coconut oil, peanuts, and salt until well coated.

Transfer to a rimmed baking sheet and roast in the oven for about 15 minutes or until fragrant.

Transfer the roasted peanuts to a bowl and add vinegar, chili powder and lime zest.

Toss to coat well and serve.

Nutritional Information per Serving:

Calories: 447; Total Fat: 39.5g; Carbs: 12.3 g; Dietary Fiber: 6.5 g; Sugars: 3 g; Protein: 18.9 g; Cholesterol: 0 mg; Sodium: 956 mg

97.Healthy Seed Crackers

Yield: 6 Servings
Total Time: 1 Hour 5 Minutes
Prep Time: 5 Minutes
Cook Time: 1 Hour

Ingredients
- 1 teaspoon sea salt
- 1/2 cup raw buckwheat
- 1/2 cup linseeds
- 1 1/2 cups sunflower seeds
- 1/4 cup chia seeds
- 1 1/2 cups warm water

Directions

Mix together all ingredients in a large bowl; set aside for about 20 minutes, stirring occasionally.
Preheat oven to 325°F.
Press the mixture into a baking tray lined with baking paper and bake for about 1 hours or until golden and crisp. Remove from oven and cut into pieces. Enjoy!

Nutritional Information per Serving:

Calories: 199; Total Fat: 12.1 g; Carbs: 16.9 g; Dietary Fiber: 8 g; Sugars: 0.3 g; Protein: 7.4 g; Cholesterol: 0 mg; Sodium: 321 mg

Yield: 3 Servings
Total Time: 55 Minutes
Prep Time: 10 Minutes
Cook Time: 45 Minutes

Ingredients:

- 1 pound fresh carrots, sliced
- 3 tablespoons sesame oil
- 2 tablespoon sesame seeds
- Pinch of sea salt
- Pinch of pepper

Directions:

Spread carrots in a baking tray and drizzle with 2 tablespoons of sesame oil and toss to coat well; bake, covered, at 400°F for about 30 minutes. Remove from oven and drizzle with remaining sesame oil; sprinkle with salt and pepper and continue baking for about 15 more minutes. Serve sprinkled with toasted sesame seeds. Enjoy!

Nutrition Information per Serving:

Calories: 217; Total Fat: 16.6 g; Carbs: 16.3 g; Dietary Fiber: 4.4 g; Sugars: 7.5 g Protein: 2.3 g; Cholesterol: 0 mg; Sodium: 183 mg

99.Sugar-Free Peanut Butter Fudge

Yield: 12 Servings
Total Time: 7 Minutes
Prep Time: 5 Minutes
Cook Time: 2 Minutes

Ingredients
- 1/4 cup vanilla almond milk
- 1 cup coconut oil
- 1 cup peanut butter

Optional Topping:
- 2 tablespoons melted coconut oil
- 1/4 cup unsweetened cocoa powder
- 2 tablespoons Swerve

Directions

Melt coconut oil and peanut butter over low heat; transfer to a blender along with the remaining ingredients and blend until very smooth.
Pour the mixture to a loaf pan lined with parchment paper. Whisk the topping ingredients in a bowl and drizzle over the fudge. Freeze until firm and serve.

Nutritional Information per Serving:

Calories: 287; Total Fat: 29.7 g; Carbs: 4 g; Dietary Fiber: 1.7 g; Sugars: 0.7 g; Protein: 5.4 g; Cholesterol: 0 mg; Sodium: 4 mg

100.Bacon-Avocado stuffed Peppers

Yield: 4 Servings
Total Time: 30 Minutes
Prep Time: 10 Minutes
Cook Time: 20 Minutes

Ingredients
- 450g sweet baby peppers
- 150g bacon, chopped
- 2 ripe avocados
- 1 tbsp. hot sauce
- 2 tbsp. freshly squeezed lime juice
- ½ bunch cilantro, chopped
- Coarse sea salt

Directions

Preheat your oven to 350 F.
Cut the peppers in half, lengthwise, removing the seeds and membrane. Arrange them in a baking sheet and lightly spray with cooking spray and bake for 10 minutes.

As the peppers are baking, mash up the avocado in a bowl and combine with the lime juice, hot sauce, salt and the cilantro and sauté the bacon in a skillet until they become crisp and browned.
Use a spoon to scoop the avocado mash into the peppers and top with bacon bits. Enjoy!

Nutritional Information per Serving:

Calories: 431; Total Fat: 35.5 g; Carbs: 17.5 g; Dietary Fiber: 8.7 g; Sugars: 3.3 g; Protein: 16.8 g; Cholesterol: 41 mg; Sodium: 971 mg

101.Tasty Coconut Raspberry Fat Bombs

Yield: 12 Servings
Total Time: 10 Minutes
Prep Time: 10 Minutes
Cook Time: N/A

Ingredients
- 1/2 cup freeze dried raspberries
- 1/2 cup coconut butter
- 1/2 cup coconut oil
- 1/2 cup unsweetened shredded coconut
- 1/4 cup powdered Swerve Sweetener
- 1 scoop protein powder

Directions

Line an 8 by 8-inch square pan with baking paper and set aside.
Grind dried berries in a food processor until fine; set aside.

In a saucepan, stir together shredded coconut, coconut oil, coconut butter, and stevia until melted and combined; pour half of the mixture into the pan and stir the ground raspberry and protein powder to the remaining mixture until well combined. Scoop raspberry mixture over the coconut mixture in pan and swirl. Freeze until firm and then cut into chunks to serve.

Nutritional Information per Serving:

Calories: 184; Total Fat: 17.9 g; Carbs: 4.3 g; Dietary Fiber: 2.7 g; Sugars: 1.3 g; Protein: 12.8 g; Cholesterol: 5 mg; Sodium: 10 mg

Yield: 20 Cookies
Total Time: 12 Minutes
Prep Time: 2 Minutes
Cook Time: 10 Minutes

Ingredients

- 3 cups finely shredded coconut flakes
- 1 cup melted coconut oil
- 1 teaspoon liquid stevia

Directions

Combine all ingredients in a large bowl; stir until well blended. Form the mixture into small balls and arrange them on a paper-lined baking tray. Press each cookie down with a fork and refrigerate until firm. Enjoy!

Nutritional Information per Serving:

Calories: 99; Total Fat: 10 g; Carbs: 2 g; Dietary Fiber: 2 g; Sugars: 0 g; Protein: 3 g; Cholesterol: 0 mg; Sodium: 7 mg

103.Cashew Butter Fat Bombs

Yield: 12 Fat Bombs
Total Time: 25 Minutes
Prep Time: 25 Minutes
Cook Time: N/A

Ingredients

- 6 tablespoons cashew butter
- 6 tablespoons grass-fed butter
- ½ teaspoon liquid stevia
- 1 teaspoon vanilla extract
- 1 pinch sea salt

Directions

Prepare mini muffin tin by lining with liners; set aside.
In a microwave safe bowl, mix grass-fed butter and cashew butter and then microwave for minute or until melted. Stir in the remaining ingredients until well blended. Spoon the mixture into the prepared muffin tin and freeze for at least 10 minute or until firm. Enjoy!

Nutritional Information per Serving

Calories: 206; Total Fat: 20 g; Carbs: 5 g; Dietary fiber: 0.5 g; Sugars: 1.6 g; Protein: 2.1 g; Cholesterol: 31 mg; Sodium: 164 mg

Printed in Great Britain
by Amazon